DEVELOPMENTAL DISEASES OF THE HIP - DIAGNOSIS AND MANAGEMENT

Edited by **Dusko Spasovski**

Developmental Diseases of the Hip - Diagnosis and Management
http://dx.doi.org/10.5772/62934
Edited by Dusko Spasovski

Contributors
Özgür Korkmaz, Melih Malkoc, Ismet Gavrankapetanovic, Adnan Papovic, Veronika Kralj-Iglič, Chunho Chen, Tingming Wang, Ken N Kuo, Maximilian Kasparek, Friedrich Boettner, Dusko Spasovski

Published by InTech
Janeza Trdine 9, 51000 Rijeka, Croatia

Publishing Process Manager Edi Lipovic
Technical Editor SPi Global
Cover InTech Design team

First published April, 2017
Printed in Croatia
Legal deposit, Croatia: National and University Library in Zagreb

Additional hard copies can be obtained from orders@intechopen.com

Developmental Diseases of the Hip - Diagnosis and Management, Edited by Dusko Spasovski
p. cm.
Print ISBN 978-953-51-3073-4
Online ISBN 978-953-51-3074-1

For EU product safety concerns:
IN TECH d.o.o., Prolaz Marije Krucifikse Kozulić 3, 51000 Rijeka, Croatia,
info@intechopen.com or visit our website at intechopen.com.

Meet the editor

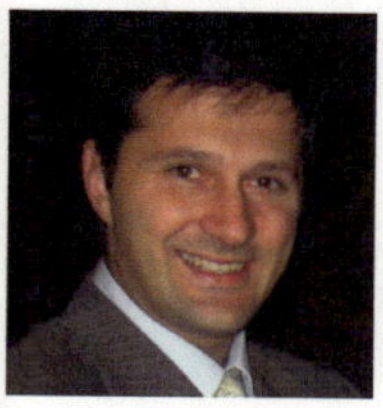

Duško Spasovski is an orthopaedic surgeon at the Institute for Orthopaedic Surgery 'Banjica' in Belgrade, Serbia. His clinical work covers paediatric orthopaedics and trauma, with recent research interests mostly in the fields of biomechanics, orthopaedic genetics and stem cell treatment in orthopaedic surgery. He is a member of the Cathedra for Surgery and Anaesthesiology at the School of Medicine, University of Belgrade. Parallel to medical studies, he graduated at the Faculty of Sports and Physical Education, and his teaching topics include various aspects of sports-related kinesiology and orthopaedics. He is very active in Dragon Boat, a competing member of the Serbian national team.

Contents

Preface

The complexity of human locomotor system generally prevents the use of analytical scientific approach: there are no 'important' and 'less important' parts. But if we were allowed to choose one that would best reflect both the paradigm of orthopaedic surgery 'Motion is life' and the amount of effort invested in achieving it, it would probably be the hip joint affected by developmental dysplasia.

There is a long list of diseases and traumatic events that affect this large joint, but none is as persistent, as elusive and with profound consequences as this condition. For many centuries, we have been struggling with the consequences while trying to understand the reasons how and why such a stable spherical joint eventually becomes dysfunctional and how to prevent it. Some of the greatest achievements in operative orthopaedics have been introduced in the effort to treat developmental dysplasia of the hip. On the other hand, implementation of diagnostic ultrasound in clinical paediatric and orthopaedic practice has significantly improved the efficacy and precision of nonoperative treatment in early childhood.

With a glimpse of new paradigm shift on a horizon (genetic testing, stem cell treatment, artificial cartilage-like biomaterials etc.) his would probably be one of the last books that describe developmental dysplasia of the hip as a challenge still not completely conquered, that we manage by predominantly major surgical interventions. From that point of view, we present an overview of contemporary approach to developmental dysplasia of the hip, covering various clinically relevant aspects in six chapters:

- Introduction to historical, demographic and socioeconomic aspects of the disease worldwide
- Biomechanical parameters of dysplastic hip joint
- Nonoperative treatment of developmental dysplasia of the hip in early childhood
- Operative procedures for correcting hip dysplasia in childhood
- Total hip replacement as a standard procedure for the management of hip dysplasia sequelae in adulthood
- Specific considerations in operative endoprosthetic reconstruction of dysplastic hips

We believe that this book will be a valuable reference to students, orthopaedic surgeons, researchers and other healthcare professionals interested in orthopaedic surgery, biomechanics and epidemiology.

I am very grateful to all the authors for their strong effort and patience needed to bring out this book. In addition, I deeply appreciate the assistance of Mr. Edi Lipović, whose guidance and encouragement were truly invaluable.

Duško Spasovski, MD, PhD
Orthopaedic Surgeon
Paediatric Orthopaedics Department, Institute for Orthopaedic Surgery 'Banjica',
Clinical Assistant at the School of Medicine, University of Belgrade, Serbia

Chapter 1

Introductory Chapter: Five-Dimensional Approach to the Developmental Dysplasia of the Hip

Duško Spasovski

Additional information is available at the end of the chapter

http://dx.doi.org/10.5772/67658

Developmental dysplasia of the hip (DDH) is not a specific disorder; it is rather a scale of overlapping and transforming conditions. It ranges from occult dysplasia seen on ultrasound screening of newborns, neonatal hip instability and dislocated hip whether reducible by orthopaedic manipulation or not. The hallmark of DDH is acetabular dysplasia—abnormality in size, shape or orientation of acetabulum. A thoughtful elucidation regarding DDH is that it is 'a common and preventable cause of childhood disability' [1]. Complications and consequences of DDH make this time interval much longer, though.

The incidence of many faces of DDH is fortunately distributed: it is reported to be as much as 8% for dysplasia, 1–3% for neonatal hip instability and <0.2% for frank dislocation [2–4]. These epidemiological data are greatly influenced by both diagnostic criteria and diagnostic methods used [5, 6]. They evolve not only due to demographic changes of population, predominantly through migrations and genetic mixing, but also due to changes in nutrition [7–9].

DDH is not a disease of modern age. It was recognised and described by Hippocrates as a congenital dislocation of the hip. Dysplastic hips and presence of false acetabulum were found in skeletons from medieval times [10–14].

Present etiological concept of DDH is multifactorial, consisting of endogenous (genetic disorders of collagen or collagen-related enzymes, transmembrane G-protein) [15, 16] and exogenous factors (related to intrauterine biomechanics, such as breech position and history of prior pregnancies, or environmental like birth in a certain season, swaddling technique) [17–19]. Breech presentation, positive family history of DDH, female sex, vaginal delivery, primiparity and oligohydramnion are usually regarded to as DDH risk factors. Some authors include other mechanical intrauterine restrictions (large baby, multiple pregnancy), advanced maternal age and delivery-related conditions (post-maturity) [1, 20]. It is worth noting that premature birth is not a risk factor for DDH [21]. Risk factors have limited clinical importance, however, due to both low sensitivity (10–27% of all infants who have DDH also have any risk factor) and low specificity (under 10% of children with risk factors have DDH) [22, 23].

Historically, there were several crucial events that improved both the diagnosing and treating this disease.

- First, understanding the hip biomechanics, Lorenz in 1895 introduced first successful method of closed reduction, using plaster cast in extreme abduction for retention [24]. Results were immediately supported with new method discovered same year: X-rays, and so the Lorenz method became widespread.
- Then, in 1935, Italian paediatrician Ortolani established a diagnostic manoeuvre used to verify present dislocation with audible and sensible 'click' [25]. He was the first to recognize the importance of diagnosis of dislocated hip in infants. A systematic screening of newborn hips has started.
- In 1944, Pavlik begun applying the harness as means for keeping dysplastic hips mobile but limited to advantageous abduction angles, thus promoting biomechanical stimulation of normal hip development [26].
- Modern operative treatment of acetabular dysplasia begun with Chiari [27] and Salter [28] pelvic osteotomy.
- In 1961, Charnley introduced modern concept of total hip replacement in the treatment of osteoarthritis, a common sequela of hip dysplasia in adult age [29].
- Following the technological improvements, Graf introduced ultrasound as a method for visualisation of the hip and described diagnostic criteria for assessment of hip dysplasia [30].
- Finally, with screening data available, Klisic introduced a new name 'developmental dysplasia' [31].

Basically, there are five very important dilemmas that demarcate the struggle with this rather recalcitrant medical condition. Their analysis reflects both the complexity of problem and diversity of solutions currently available across the medical practice in the whole world.

1. Screening for hip dysplasia: overlooking versus overtreating

Neonatal hip joint demonstrates significant potential for growth and remodelling. Still, the outcome of nonoperative reduction of dislocated femoral head and its safe containment within the acetabulum strongly depends on timing. If a treatment begins within first 7 weeks, it will be highly successful [32–35] regardless if one or both hips are treated [36]. That is why meticulous clinical examination of hips in newborns is mandatory for decades. Establishing a diagnosis of DDH after 3 months of age is considered as a late presentation, with estimated incidence from 0.02 to 0.2% [37, 38]. It is associated with higher rate of operative treatment, worse prognosis and increased healthcare cost [39–43].

Unstable or dislocated hip is usually diagnosed by combined Ortolani-Barlow manoeuvre, with satisfactory specificity (>84%) but controversial sensitivity (from 7 to 98% in various studies) [44]. These clinical signs, however, cannot pinpoint acetabular dysplasia. For that reason, in some medical systems, an ultrasound screening is also mandatory and universal [8], while in others, it is used only in selected, targeted cases [45]. These variations in screening protocol are due to economic, organisational reasons, as well as the concern of over diagnosing and possible unnecessary treatment [46–48]. Most common ultrasound screening methods are according to Graf, Harcke, Terjesen and Suzuki. Data from Austria, UK and Ireland suggest that universal ultrasonic screening for DDH reduced both overall average healthcare expenses and the need for operative treatment [2, 45, 49–52], although there are different opinions in the USA [53].

While very valuable for early detection of hip dislocation, and without any absolute contraindications [54] ultrasound in first 2 weeks of life has limited sensitivity to detect clinically relevant dysplasia, since a fraction of newborns have underdeveloped but healthy hips—a temporarily false positive result [4, 55, 56]. Some authors even suggest that ultrasound in first 6 weeks should confirm the diagnosis of DDH only if hip is decentred (Graf III type) or dislocated (Graf IV type). For true incidence of hip dysplasia, a correlation of ultrasound data, clinical examination and the number of late presented cases requiring operative treatment should all be analysed.

Nevertheless, the problem how to discriminate between dysplastic hips and healthy hips still remains—ultrasound is too dependent on examiner's skills, while radiographic criteria are usually biased by pelvic rotation [57]. Effective screening for DDH should be characterised by low percentage of cases that require surgical intervention, and all of those due to failures of nonoperative treatment, rather than due to late detection [49, 58]. In some studies, the majority of patients with symptomatic dysplasia in adult age did not meet criteria for selective ultrasound screening in infant age—they were false negative on clinical examination [59].

2. Neonatal hip instability: nature versus therapy

Like hip dysplasia, neonatal hip instability follows similar diagnostic concerns. This condition is diagnosed either by provocative tests (Barlow) or by dynamic ultrasound testing (Harcke technique) [60] with substantial reproducibility and accuracy only achieved in combination of these methods [40]. On the other hand, failure of recognition and treatment of neonatal hip instability can lead to significant hip dysfunction [61].

Neonates are usually born with slight flexion contracture (25–30°), which should spontaneously decrease to <20° at 6 weeks, and 7° at 12 weeks. In addition, one should bear in mind that majority of hips clinically unstable at birth will resolve spontaneously within first 8 weeks [62], in some cases until 3 years of age [63]. In other words, specificity of clinical and ultrasonic examination improves with growth. This is particularly true for testing if there is limited abduction, which meets its peak of reliability as DDH marker at the age between 3 and 6 months [64].

The relation between abduction position and movements and proper stimulation of dysplastic/unstable acetabulum to become better is clearly demonstrated, and positioning of legs influences the outcome of hip development [65]. While wide (double) diapering stimulates beneficial dynamic abduction of both hips, there is also an opposite praxis of swaddling (hips in extension and in zero abduction) either due to traditional routine in some parts of the world (Middle East, Japan, Native Americans, etc.) [66–68] or for the prevention of excessive crying and promoting sleep [69]. It is clear, however, that risk for hip deterioration if legs are kept laced grossly surpasses all potential benefits, which are easily achievable by other, less hazardous means.

3. Natural history of DDH: prevention versus operation

We already stated that dysplastic and unstable hips may undergo spontaneous recovery [70]. As for the cohort of non-recovering hips, it has been observed that DDH leads to significant loss of normal joint function [71]. Dysplastic hips have tendency to evolve over years into painful and debilitating osteoarthritis [72–74], while dislocated hips are accompanied with short posture and waddling gait throughout life, and if not reduced operatively within the first 8 years, painful syndrome may eventually develop [59, 75]. In patients with untreated unilateral dislocation, pelvic obliquity deteriorates the distribution of hip force on contralateral hip joint, contributing to degeneration on that side as well, along with further compensatory dysfunctions of trunk and knees [11].

DDH and osteoarthritis share genetic biomechanical etiological aspects [76]. Longitudinal studies have revealed that degenerative changes induced by hip dysplasia develop more rapidly than in other predisposing conditions [77]. Total hip replacement (THR) is a surgical procedure that is most often performed in treating symptomatic advanced osteoarthritis, especially in younger age [78–82]. The diagnosis of DDH in first-order relative increases a chance for THR by the age of 65 [83]. Recent studies show that average hospital cost for primary THR secondary to DDH is higher than in other cases. Also, the severity of DDH additionally increases those expenses [79, 84]. If DDH is diagnosed early and the treatment was nonoperative, the rate of osteoarthritis at long-term follow-up is twice lower than after open reduction [81]. On the other hand, survival rate of dislocated hips that undergone operative treatment in infancy including innominate osteotomy was 54% at the age of 45 [85].

4. The follow-up challenge: hip morphology versus function

Since DDH is a kind of 'moving target' throughout patient's life, several assessment protocols are in use for follow-up once the diagnosis is established, depending on the kind of intervention (observation, nonoperative or operative procedure), age and complaints. They all have the same two prominent characteristics:

(a) Low reliability and inter-observer concordance [86].

(b) Inadequate correlation of functional and radiographic results [87], implying that not all radiographically dysplastic/arthritic hip joints are the same, and that more than morphologic factors influence the onset and severity of symptoms.

Health-related part of elusive term we refer to as 'quality of life' (QoL) includes, but is not limited to, satisfaction in physical, emotional and social aspects of life. Quality of life with DDH is mostly affected by pain, gait disturbance, limited range of motion and leg length discrepancy. These factors are not independent, they aggravate each other. Patients become regular consumers of various healthcare services and products, spending days and money on rehabilitation, usually getting weight because of inadequate activity. Several studies demonstrated long-term improvement in QoL after THA in patients diagnosed with DDH [88, 89]. Although very important for patient, QoL assessment should be primarily used to identify their expectation regarding the type of treatment and should not replace clinical examination and standard diagnostic methods [90, 91].

5. The impact of DDH on healthcare: cause versus effect

Many diseases have been imposing a strong burden to healthcare service on global scale, in aspects of organisation, cost and consequences of diagnostic and therapeutic modalities indicated. In a rather long list, one could count in tuberculosis, diabetes, cardiac failure, cancer, AiDS and DDH. Most of them share the same characteristic of significant mortality, direct or indirect through complications. On the other hand, DDH is among the few exceptions that are not directly life threatening but deteriorate the quality of life and/or working ability up to great extent and for a long time [92].

Osteoarthritis is one of the major causes of non-cancer pain, impairing daily and social activities, and carrying a significant economic burden measurable in billions of dollars annually [93, 94]. Estimations are that there are more than 4.7 million THA operations done annually in the whole world, with significant portion due to DDH [95]. Average total expenses of THA treatment are about 20,000 euros per patient [17], with great variance. For illustration, in Serbian healthcare system, it is less than 10,000 euros using the same modern implants.

In accordance to non-maleficent approach, detailed patient examination and utilisation of all diagnostic and therapeutic procedures that are indicated for suspected condition in every patient, always leads to better clinical outcome. But in everyday practice, there is usually more than one option for every step in patient management. These options sometimes differ not only in side effects, reliability, safety or indication requirements but also in technical and financial availability. That's where statistics and economics come to interfere with strictly medical issues. In some cases, such as DDH, many factors need to be considered in order to see the whole picture [96–98].

For instance, introduction of ultrasound examination to clinical screening for hip dysplasia revealed that some clinically positive cases are false positive, but also vice versa; it brought a fraction of clinically normal, but sonographically dysplastic or lax hips. Since it incurred extra cost and organisational effort, subsequent justification had to come from economic studies [45, 68].

Factors that contribute to late diagnosing of DDH include inconsistent implementation of screening protocol, lack of appropriate awareness of the disease and its complications and insufficient training in proper and timely detection of DDH and therapeutic actions [42, 99]. Important but often neglected issue in this situation, where operative treatment makes the method of choice, is the involvement of parents (usually mother) in the process of treatment. Mothers stay with their child for the whole duration of the treatment—usually for 3–6 months following open reduction, with the child immobilised in bed by plaster cast or skin traction, in hospital and/or at home for weeks. This is tangled with many new problems involving the patient itself (such as feeding, hygiene in the cast, dressing, sleeping, transport), mother (employment status, social isolation, existing physical and mental health condition) and the rest of the family (altered daily activities) for a long period of time [100]. There is a general lack of information and outpatient support about recovering child's complex needs during that period [101, 102].

Summary

There is considerable diversity in opinions worldwide regarding both diagnostic and therapeutic approach to DDH. Besides orthopaedic, many other factors could contribute to it: demographic, socioeconomic and differences regarding healthcare organisation [5]. Reflecting this diversity, in this book authors will present their experience and opinion on several important issues regarding DDH: screening for DDH, biomechanical considerations, diagnostic procedures in all age groups, treatment modalities of hip dysplasia and dislocation in childhood, and dealing with the consequences in adulthood.

Author details

Duško Spasovski

Address all correspondence to: duskosp@gmail.com

Paediatric Orthopaedics Department, Institute for Orthopaedic Surgery "Banjica", Belgrade, Serbia

School of Medicine, University of Belgrade, Serbia

References

[1] Woodacre T, Ball T, Cox P. Epidemiology of developmental dysplasia of the hip within the UK: refining the risk factors. Journal of Children's Orthopaedics. 2016;10(6):633–42.

[2] Woodacre T, Dhadwal A, Ball T, Edwards C, Cox PJ. The costs of late detection of developmental dysplasia of the hip. Journal of Children's Orthopaedics. 2014;8(4):325–32.

[3] Jacobsen S, Sonne-Holm S, Søballe K, Gebuhr P, Lund B. Hip dysplasia and osteoarthrosis: a survey of 4151 subjects from the Osteoarthrosis Substudy of the Copenhagen City Heart Study. Acta Orthopaedica. 2005;76(2):149–58.

[4] Dezateux C, Rosendahl K. Developmental dysplasia of the hip. Lancet. 2007;369(9572): 1541–52.

[5] Mulpuri K, Schaeffer EK, Kelley SP, Castañeda P, Clarke NM, Herrera-Soto JA, Upasani V, Narayanan UG, Price CT, IHDI Study Group. What is the impact of center variability in a multicenter international prospective observational study on developmental dysplasia of the hip? Clinical Orthopaedics and Related Research. 2016;474(5):1138–45.

[6] Dogruel H, Atalar H, Yavuz OY, Sayli U. Clinical examination versus ultrasonography in detecting developmental dysplasia of the hip. International Orthopaedics. 2008;32:415–9.

[7] Loder RT, Shafer C. The demographics of developmental hip dysplasia in the Midwestern United States (Indiana). Journal of Children's Orthopaedics. 2015;9(1):93–8.

[8] Thaler M, Biedermann R, Lair J, et al. Cost-effectiveness of universal ultrasound screening compared with clinical examination alone in the diagnosis and treatment of neonatal hip dysplasia in Austria. The Journal of Bone and Joint Surgery. British Volume. 2011;93:1126–30.

[9] Grundt JH, Nakling J, Eide GE, Markestad T. Possible relation between maternal consumption of added sugar and sugar-sweetened beverages and birth weight—time trends in a population. BMC Public Health. 2012;12:901.

[10] Rogers J, Watt I, Dieppe P. Medical history: arthritis in Saxon and mediaeval skeletons. BMJ. 1981;283(6307):1668–70.

[11] Loder RT, Skopelja EN. The epidemiology and demographics of hip dysplasia. ISRN Orthopedics. 2011:1-46.

[12] Thould AK, Thould BT. Arthritis in Roman Britain. BMJ. 1983;287(6409):1909–11.

[13] Blatt SH. To swaddle, or not to swaddle? Paleoepidemiology of developmental dysplasia of the hip and the swaddling dilemma among the indigenous populations of North America. American Journal of Human Biology. 2015;27(1):116–28.

[14] Mitchell PD, Redfern RC. Diagnostic criteria for developmental dislocation of the hip in human skeletal remains. International Journal of Osteoarchaeology. 2008;18(1):61–71.

[15] Soran N, Altindag O, Aksoy N, Cakır H, Taşkın A, Soran M, Işıkan E. The association of serum prolidase activity with developmental dysplasia of the hip. Rheumatology International. 2013;33(8):1939–42.

[16] Feldman GJ, Parvizi J, Levenstien M et al. Developmental dysplasia of the hip: linkage mapping and whole exome sequencing identify a shared variant in CX3CR1 in all affected members of a large multigeneration family. Journal of Bone and Mineral Research. 2013;28:2540–9.

[17] Palmén K. Prevention of congenital dislocation of the hip. Acta Orthopaedica Scandinavica. 1984;55(208):5–107.

[18] Loder RT, Shafer C. Seasonal variation in children with developmental dysplasia of the hip. Journal of Children's Orthopaedics. 2014;8(1):11–22.

[19] Colta RC, Stoicanescu C, Nicolae M, Oros S, Burnei G. Hip dysplasia screening-epidemiological data from Valcea County. Journal of Medicine and Life. 2016;9(1):106.

[20] Chan A, McCaul K, Cundy P, Haan E, Byron-Scott R. Perinatal risk factors for developmental dysplasia of the hip. Archives of Disease in Childhood. Fetal and Neonatal Edition. 1997;76(2):F94–100.

[21] Orak MM, Onay T, Gümüştaş SA, Gürsoy T, Muratlí HH. Is prematurity a risk factor for developmental dysplasia of the hip? A prospective study. The Bone & Joint Journal. 2015;97(B):716–20.

[22] Boere-Boonekamp MM, Kerkhoff TH, Schuil PB, et al. Early detection of developmental dysplasia of the hip in The Netherlands: the validity of a standardized assessment protocol in infants. American Journal of Public Health. 1998;88(2):285–8.

[23] Sahin F, Akturk A, Beyazova U, et al. Screening for developmental dysplasia of the hip: results of a 7-year follow-up study. Pediatrics International. 2004;46(2):162-6.

[24] Lorenz A. The So-Called Congenital Dislocation of the Hip. Its Pathology and Treatment. Stuttgart: Enke; 1920, pp. 95–6.

[25] Ortolani M. A very little known sign and its importance in the early diagnosis of congenital hip predislocation. Pediatria. 1937;45:129.

[26] Pavlik A. Method of functional therapy with strap braces as a principle of conservative therapy of congenital dislocation of the hip in infants. Zeitschrift fur Orthopadie and Ihre Grenzgebiete. 1957;89:341–52.

[27] Chiari K. Results of pelvic osteotomy as of the shelf method acetabular roof plastic. Zeitschrift fur Orthopadie and Ihre Grenzgebiete. 1955;87(1):14–26.

[28] Salter RB. Innominate osteotomy in the treatment of congenital dislocation and subluxation of the hip. The Bone & Joint Journal. 1961;43(3):518–39.

[29] Charnley J. Arthroplasty of the hip: a new operation. Lancet. 1961;1(7187):1129–32.

[30] Graf R. The diagnosis of congenital hip-joint dislocation by the ultrasound combound treatment. Archives of Orthopaedic and Trauma Surgery. 1980;97:117–33.

[31] Klisic PJ. Congenital dislocation of the hip: a misleading term. The Journal of Bone and Joint Surgery. British Volume. 1989;71:136.

[32] Van der Sluijs JA, De Gier L, Verbeke JI et al. Prolonged treatment with the Pavlik harness in infants with developmental dysplasia of the hip. The Journal of Bone and Joint Surgery. British Volume. 2009;91:1090–3.

[33] Atalar H, Sayli U, Yavuz OY, Uras I, Dogruel H. Indicators of successful use of the Pavlik harness in infants with developmental dysplasia of the hip. International Orthopaedics. 2007;31:145–50.

[34] Walton MJ, Isaacson Z, McMillan D, Hawkes R, Atherton WG. The success of management with the Pavlik harness for developmental dysplasia of the hip using a United Kingdom screening programme and ultrasound-guided supervision. The Journal of Bone and Joint Surgery. British Volume. 2010;92:1013–16.

[35] Cashman JP, Round J, Taylor G, Clarke NM. The natural history of developmental dysplasia of the hip after early supervised treatment in the Pavlik harness. A prospective, longitudinal follow-up. The Journal of Bone and Joint Surgery. British Volume. 2002;84:418–25.

[36] Borowski A, Thawrani D, Grissom L, Littleton AG, Thacker MM. Bilaterally dislocated hips treated with the Pavlik harness are not at a higher risk for failure. Journal of Pediatric Orthopaedics. 2009;29:661–5.

[37] Azzopardi T, van Essen P, Cundy P, Tucker G, Chan A. Late diagnosis of developmental dysplasia of the hip: an analysis of risk factors. Journal of Pediatric Orthopaedics B. 2011;20:1–7.

[38] Pollet V, Percy V, Prior HJ. Relative risk and incidence for developmental dysplasia of the hip. The Journal of Pediatrics. 2016;181:202-7.

[39] Sharpe P, Mulpuri K, Chan A, Cundy PJ. Differences in risk factors between early and late diagnosed developmental dysplasia of the hip. Archives of Disease in Childhood. Fetal and Neonatal Edition. 2006;91(3):158–62.

[40] American Academy of Paediatrics. Committee on Quality Improvement, Subcommittee on Developmental Dysplasia of the Hip. Clinical practice guideline: early detection of developmental dysplasia of the hip. Pediatrics. 2000;105:896.

[41] Sewell MD, Eastwood DM. Screening and treatment in developmental dysplasia of the hip-where do we go from here? International Orthopaedics. 2011;35(9):1359–67.

[42] Yagmurlu MF, Bayhan IA, Tuhanioglu U, Kilinc AS, Karakas ES. Clinical and radiological outcomes are correlated with the age of the child in single-stage surgical treatment of developmental dysplasia of the hip. Acta Orthopaedica Belgica. 2013;79(2):159–65.

[43] Studer K, Williams N, Antoniou G, Gibson C, Scott H, Scheil WK, Foster BK, Cundy PJ. Increase in late diagnosed developmental dysplasia of the hip in South Australia: risk factors, proposed solutions. Medical Journal of Australia. 2016;204(6):240.

[44] Omeroglu H, Koparal S. The role of clinical examination and risk factors in the diagnosis of developmental dysplasia of the hip: a prospective study in 188 referred infants. Archives of Orthopaedic and Trauma Surgery. 2001;121:7–11.

[45] Elbourne D, Dezateux C, Arthur R, Clarke NM, Gray A, King A, Quinn A, Gardner F, Russell G. Ultrasonography in the diagnosis and management of developmental hip dysplasia (UK Hip Trial): clinical and economic results of a multicentre randomised controlled trial. Lancet. 2002;360(9350):2009–17.

[46] Phelan N, Thoren J, Fox C, O'Daly BJ, O'Beirne J. Developmental dysplasia of the hip: incidence and treatment outcomes in the Southeast of Ireland. Irish Journal of Medical Science. 2015;184(2):411–5.

[47] von Kries Reudiger, et al. General ultrasound screening reduces the rate of first operative procedures for developmental dysplasia of the hip: a case-control study. The Journal of Pediatrics. 2012;160(2):271–5.

[48] Lennox IAC, McLauchlan J, Murali R. Failures of screening and management of congenital dislocation of the hip. The Journal of Bone and Joint Surgery. 1993;75-B:72–5.

[49] Clegg J, Bache CE, Raut VV. Financial justification for routine ultrasound screening of the neonatal hip. The Journal of Bone and Joint Surgery. British Volume. 1999;81-B:852–7.

[50] Gray A, Elbourne D, Dezateux C, King A, Quinn A, Gardner F, United Kingdom Collaborative Hip Trial Group. Economic evaluation of ultrasonography in the diagnosis and management of developmental hip dysplasia in the United Kingdom and Ireland. The Journal of Bone and Joint Surgery. American Volume. 2005;87(11):2472–9.

[51] Thallinger C, Pospischill R, Ganger R, Radler C, Krall C, Grill F. Long-term results of a nationwide general ultrasound screening system for developmental disorders of the hip: the Austrian hip screening program. Journal of Children's Orthopaedics. 2014;8(1):3–10.

[52] Kolb A, Schweiger N, Mailath-Pokorny M, Kaider A, Hobusch G, Chiari C, Windhager R. Low incidence of early developmental dysplasia of the hip in universal ultrasonographic screening of newborns: analysis and evaluation of risk factors. International Orthopaedics. 2016;40(1):123–7.

[53] US Preventive Services Task Force. Screening for developmental dysplasia of the hip: recommendation statement. Pediatrics. 2006;117(3):898–902.

[54] American Institute of Ultrasound in Medicine. AIUM practice guideline for the performance of an ultrasound examination for detection and assessment of developmental dysplasia of the hip. Journal of Ultrasound in Medicine. 2009;28:114–9.

[55] Delaney LR, Karmazyn B. Developmental dysplasia of the hip: background and the utility of ultrasound. Seminars in Ultrasound, CT and MRI. 2011;32(2):151–6.

[56] Gardner R, Alshryda S, Kelley SP, Wedge J. Evidence-based management of developmental dysplasia of the hip. In: Alshryda S, Huntley J, Banaszkiewicz PA, editors. Paediatric orthopaedics: an evidenced-based approach to clinical questions. Springer; Basel, Switzerland;2016, pp. 27–42.

[57] Wenger D, Düppe H, Tiderius CJ. Acetabular dysplasia at the age of 1 year in children with neonatal instability of the hip: a cohort study of 243 infants. Acta Orthopaedica. 2013;84(5):483–8.

[58] Sanghrajka AP, Murnaghan CF, Shekkeris A, Eastwood DM. Open reduction for developmental dysplasia of the hip: failures of screening or failures of treatment? The Annals of the Royal College of Surgeons of England. 2013;95(2):113–7.

[59] Sink EL, Ricciardi BF, Torre KD, Price CT. Selective ultrasound screening is inadequate to identify patients who present with symptomatic adult acetabular dysplasia. Journal of Children's Orthopaedics. 2014;8:451–5.

[60] Harcke HT, Clarke NM, Lee MS et al. Examination of the infant hip with real-time ultrasonography. Journal of Ultrasound in Medicine. 1984;3:131–7.

[61] Engesaeter IO, Lie SA, Lehmann TG, Furnes O, Vollset SE, Engesaeter LB. Neonatal hip instability and risk of total hip replacement in young adulthood: follow-up of 2,218,596

newborns from the Medical Birth Registry of Norway in the Norwegian Arthroplasty Register. Acta Orthopaedica. 2008;79:321–6.

[62] Kotlarsky P, Haber R, Bialik V, Eidelman M. Developmental dysplasia of the hip: what has changed in the last 20 years? World Journal of Orthopedics. 2015;6(11):886.

[63] Pruszczynski B, Harcke HT, Holmes L, Bowen JR. Natural history of hip instability in infants (without subluxation or dislocation): a three year follow-up. BMC Musculoskeletal Disorders. 2014;15(1):1.

[64] Shipman SA, Helfand M, Moyer VA, Yawn BP. Screening for developmental dysplasia of the hip: a systematic literature review for the US Preventive Services Task Force. Pediatrics. 2006;117(3):e557–76.

[65] Mahan ST, Kasser JR. Does swaddling influence developmental dysplasia of the hip? Pediatrics. 2008;121:177–8.

[66] Schwend RM, Shaw BA, Segal LS. Evaluation and treatment of developmental hip dysplasia in the newborn and infant. Pediatric Clinics of North America. 2014;61:1095–107.

[67] Yamamuro T, Ishida K. Recent advances in the prevention, early diagnosis, and treatment of congenital dislocation of the hip in Japan. Clinical Orthopaedics and Related Research. 1984;184:34–40.

[68] Kutlu A, Memik R, Mutlu M, Kutlu R, Arslan A. Congenital dislocation of the hip and its relation to swaddling used in Turkey. Journal of Pediatric Orthopaedics. 1992;12:598–602.

[69] Clarke NM. Swaddling and hip dysplasia: an orthopaedic perspective. Archives of Disease in Childhood. 2014;99(1):5–6.

[70] Munkhuu B, Essig S, Renchinnyam E, Schmid R, Wilhelm C, Bohlius J, Chuluunbaatar B, Shonkhuuz E, Baumann T. Incidence and treatment of developmental hip dysplasia in Mongolia: a prospective cohort study. PLoS One. 2013;8(10):e79427.

[71] Angliss R, Fujii G, Pickvance E, Wainwright AM, Benson MKD. Surgical treatment of late developmental displacement of the hip. The Journal of Bone and Joint Surgery. British Volume. 2005;87:384–94.

[72] Murphy SB, Ganz R, Muller ME. The prognosis in untreated dysplasia of the hip. A study of radiographic factors that predict the outcome. The Journal of Bone and Joint Surgery. American Volume. 1995;77:985–9.

[73] Harris WH. Etiology of osteoarthritis of the hip. Clinical Orthopaedics and Related Research. 1986;213:20–33.

[74] Mahan ST, Katz JN, Kim YJ. To screen or not to screen? A decision analysis of the utility of screening for developmental dysplasia of the hip. The Journal of Bone and Joint Surgery. American Volume. 2009;91:1705–19.

[75] Hartofilakidis G, Lampropoulou-Adamidou K. Lessons learned from study of congenital hip disease in adults. World Journal of Orthopedics. 2016;7(12):785.

[76] Altman RD, Hochberg MC, Moskowitz RW, Schnitzer TH. Recommendations for the medical management of osteoarthritis of the hip and knee: 2000 update. Arthritis & Rheumatism. 2000;43(9):1905–15.

[77] Wyles CC, Heidenreich MJ, Jeng J, Larson DR, Trousdale RT, Sierra RJ. The John Charnley award: redefining the natural history of osteoarthritis in patients with hip dysplasia and impingement. Clinical Orthopaedics and Related Research. 2017;475(2):336-50.

[78] Engesaeter IO, Lehmann T, Laborie LB, Lie SA, Rosendahl K, Engesaeter LB. Total hip replacement in young adults with hip dysplasia: age at diagnosis, previous treatment, quality of life, and validation of diagnoses reported to the Norwegian Arthroplasty Register between 1987 and 2007. Acta Orthopaedica. 2011;82(2): 149–54.

[79] Ashraf A, Larson AN, Maradit-Kremers H, Kremers WK, Lewallen DG. Hospital costs of total hip arthroplasty for developmental dysplasia of the hip. Clinical Orthopaedics and Related Research. 2014;472(7):2237–44.

[80] Australian Orthopaedic Association. National joint replacement registry annual report. AOA, Adelaide; 2011.

[81] Swedish Hip Arthroplasty Register. Annual report 2010 Göteborg. 2011. Accessed from http://www.shpr.se/en/default.aspx

[82] National Joint Replacement Registry for England and Wales. 8th annual report 2011 Hertfordshire. 2011. Accessed from www.njrcentre.org.uk

[83] Lee CB, Mata-Fink A, Millis MB, Kim YJ. Demographic differences in adolescent-diagnosed and adult-diagnosed acetabular dysplasia compared with infantile developmental dysplasia of the hip. Journal of Pediatric Orthopaedics. 2013;33(2):107–11.

[84] Sakellariou VI, Christodoulou M, Sasalos G, Babis GC. Reconstruction of the acetabulum in developmental dysplasia of the hip in total hip replacement. The Archives of Bone and Joint Surgery. 2014;2(3):130–6.

[85] Thomas SR, Wedge JH, Salter RB. Outcome at forty-five years after open reduction and innominate osteotomy for late-presenting developmental dislocation of the hip. The Journal of Bone and Joint Surgery. American Volume. 2007;89:2341–50.

[86] Ali AM, Angliss R, Fujii G, et al. Reliability of the Severin classification in the assessment of developmental dysplasia of the hip. Journal of Pediatric Orthopaedics B. 2001;10(4):293–7.

[87] Schwend RM, Pratt WB, Fultz J. Untreated acetabular dysplasia of the hip in the Navajo. A 34 year case series follow-up. Clinical Orthopaedics and Related Research. 1999;364:108–16.

[88] Knutsson S, Engberg IB. An evaluation of patients' quality of life before, 6 weeks and 6 months after total hip replacement surgery. Journal of Advanced Nursing. 1999;30(6):1349–59.

[89] Roidis NT, Pollalis AP, Hartofilakidis GC. Total hip arthroplasty in young females with congenital dislocation of the hip, radically improves their long-term quality of life. Journal of Arthroplasty. 2013;28(7):1206–11.

[90] Motamed N, Ayatollahi A, Zare N, Sadeghi Hassanabadi A. Validity and reliability of the Persian translation of the SF-36 version 2 questionnaire. Eastern Mediterranean Health Journal. 2005;11(3):349–57.

[91] Sanei F, Jamebozorgi AA, Irani A, Akbarzade Baghban A, Qoreishi M. Comparing the quality of life before and after total hip arthroplasty operation in patients with developmental dysplasia of the hip. Physical Treatments-Specific Physical Therapy Journal. 2016;5(4):219–24.

[92] World Health Organization. World report on disability. Malta: WHO; 2011. Accessed from http://www.who.int/disabilities/world_report/2011/en/ index.html

[93] Institute of Medicine. Relieving pain in America: a blueprint for transforming prevention, care, education and research. The National Academies Press, Washington, DC; 2011.

[94] Gustavsson A, Bjorkman J, Ljungcrantz C, Rhodin A, Rivano-Fischer M, Sjolund KF, et al. Socio-economic burden of patients with a diagnosis related to chronic pain-register data of 840,000 Swedish patients. European Journal of Pain. 2012;16(2):289–99.

[95] Li H, Wang L, Dai K, Zhu Z. Autogenous impaction grafting in total hip arthroplasty with developmental dysplasia of the hip. Journal of Arthroplasty. 2013;28(4):637–43.

[96] Araujo B, Hernández Simón LM, Domininguez Hernández VM. Systemic parameter estimation for the diagnosis and treatment of developmental dysplasia of the hip in children. In: Proceedings of the 58th Annual Meeting of the ISSS, Washington, DC; Vol. 1(1); 2015.

[97] Laborie LB, Engesæter IØ, Lehmann TG, Eastwood DM, Engesæter LB, Rosendahl K. Screening strategies for hip dysplasia: long-term outcome of a randomized controlled trial. Pediatrics. 2013;132:492–501.

[98] Shorter D, Hong T, Osborn DA. Cochrane review: screening programmes for developmental dysplasia of the hip in newborn infants. Evidence Based Child Health. 2013;8:11–54.

[99] Melo TE, Resende TM, Silva RC, Cruz SA, Oliveira VM. Developmental dysplasia of the hip: do the responsible for screening know what to do? Acta Ortopédica Brasileira. 2016;24(6):312–7.

[100] Demir SG, Erden S, Bulut H, Carboga B, Elbas NO. The problems experienced by parents providing postoperative home care following their child's surgery for developmental dysplasia of the hip. Orthopaedic Nursing. 2015;34(5):280–6.

[101] Sparks L, Ortman MR, Aubuchon P. Meeting the developmental needs of a child in a body cast. Journal of Orthopaedic Nursing. 2005;9(1):35–8.

[102] Tiroyan M. Investigation of obstacles for early detection of developmental dysplasia of the hip in children. Master thesis. American University of Armenia, Yerevana; 2007.

Chapter 2

Understanding Hip Biomechanics: From Simple Equilibrium to Personalized HIPSTRESS Method

Veronika Kralj-Iglič

Additional information is available at the end of the chapter

http://dx.doi.org/10.5772/66753

Abstract

It is useful to have a quantitative measure of the contact hip stress and other relevant biomechanical parameters. Parameters that correlate with clinically relevant features are sought and relations between these parameters are studied. For this purpose, two different models for the resultant hip force in the one-legged stance (the primitive model and the HIPSTRESS model) are presented with which the effect of the shape of the pelvis and proximal femora is described. Also, a special case of the primitive model—the simple balance approximation—is considered. All three descriptions are based on the equilibrium of forces of torques and differ by increasing amount of information on the shape of the particular subject. It is shown in a case of normal hip and pelvis geometry that the primitive model gives similar values of biomechanical parameters as the HIPSTRESS model that was validated by clinical studies. The primitive model (but not the simple balance approximation) merits to minimal standards to be used for understanding of the principles of the equilibrium of the forces and torques in the one-legged stance and can in certain cases (such as the one shown) also yield a valid quantitative estimation of the biomechanical parameters.

Keywords: hip stress, resultant hip force, hip osteoarthritis, cartilage degeneration, hip dysplasia, hip osteotomy

1. Equilibrium of forces and torques

Within biomechanics the effects of mechanical forces (forces due to gravity, elasticity, and friction) on living mechanisms are considered. These forces determine the movement of human and animals which is, especially in vertebrates, enabled by a complex and interconnected network of muscles, tendons, and bones that act as a consistent kinematical chain. A living system is never static on the cellular level, however, as a whole, the body can attain certain positions which are taken to correspond to static equilibria. The body is in static equilibrium when the sum of all external forces acting upon it equals to zero and sum of all torques subject to these forces equals to zero. The first condition is expressed by equation

$$\mathbf{F} = (-F \sin \vartheta_F, -F \cos \vartheta_F, 0) \tag{1}$$

where $\mathbf{F}_i = (F_{x,i}, F_{y,i}, F_{z,i})$ is the i-th force and the second condition is expressed by equation

$$\begin{aligned} \mathbf{M}_F = \mathbf{r}_F \times \mathbf{F} &= \begin{bmatrix} \mathbf{i} & \mathbf{j} & \mathbf{k} \\ -x_F & y_F & 0 \\ -F \sin \vartheta_F & -F \cos \vartheta_F & 0 \end{bmatrix} \\ &= (0, 0, x_F F \sin \vartheta_F + y_F F \cos \vartheta_F), \end{aligned} \tag{2}$$

where $\mathbf{M}_i = (M_{x,i}, M_{y,i}, M_{z,i})$ is the torque of the i-th external force, defined as a cross product

$$-x_{\text{CM}}(W_{\text{B}} - W_{\text{L}}) + F(x_F \cos \vartheta_F + y_F \sin \vartheta_F) = 0. \tag{3}$$

with $\mathbf{r}_i = (x_i, y_i, z_i)$ the momentum arm of the i-th external force. Index i runs over all forces acting upon the body.

The cross product can be expressed by the matrix

$$\mathbf{M}_i = \mathbf{r}_i \times \mathbf{F}_i = \begin{bmatrix} \mathbf{i} & \mathbf{j} & \mathbf{k} \\ x_i & y_i & z_i \\ F_{x,i} & F_{y,i} & F_{z,i} \end{bmatrix} \tag{4}$$

with the result

$$\mathbf{M}_i = \left((y_i F_{z,i} - z_i F_{y,i}), (z_i F_{x,i} - x_i F_{z,i}), (x_i F_{y,i} - y_i F_{x,i}) \right) \tag{5}$$

In the description of the static equilibrium, the image of the body is divided into segments. These segments act one upon another which is expressed by means of intersegment forces. The segments are also subjected to attraction of the Earth. As these forces and their momentum arms in general attain different directions in space, all torque components have in general nonzero values. However, in certain situations the expressions are simplified, such as in the case where the balance consists of a dimensionless rigid rod supported in a certain point, with two vertical load forces $\mathbf{F}_1$ and $\mathbf{F}_2$, each acting on a different side of the support, with momentum arms r_1 in r_2 (**Figure 1**). Let the positive x-axis point in the medial direction, positive y-axis in the superior direction, and positive z-axis in the anterior direction.

There are three forces acting on the balance, the two load forces $\mathbf{F}_1$ in $\mathbf{F}_2$ and the ground force originating in the support point. This force is called the resultant force $\mathbf{R}$. As the forces $\mathbf{F}_1$ and $\mathbf{F}_2$ act in the negative vertical direction,

$$\mathbf{F}_1 = (0, -F_1, 0), \tag{6}$$

$$\mathbf{F}_2 = (0, -F_2, 0). \tag{7}$$

The resultant force is not known; therefore, we will consider that it has three components,

$$\mathbf{R} = (R_x, R_y, R_z) \tag{8}$$

To determine the momentum arms, a choice of the origin of the coordinate system must be made. It is convenient to choose it at the origin of the resultant force **R**. In general, the momentum arms have three components,

$$\mathbf{r}_1 = (x_1, y_1, z_1) \tag{9}$$

$$\mathbf{r}_2 = (x_2, y_2, z_2) \tag{10}$$

however, in the case presented in **Figure 1**, the rod extends in the direction of x-axis only, and therefore the components of the momenta in the directions of y and z axes are equal to zero. The momentum arm of the force $\mathbf{F}_1$ points in the negative direction of x-axis,

$$\mathbf{r}_1 = (-x_1, 0, 0) \tag{11}$$

while the momentum arm of the force $\mathbf{F}_2$ points in the positive direction of x-axis,

$$\mathbf{r}_2 = (x_2, 0, 0) \tag{12}$$

The momentum arm of the resultant force **R** is zero, due to our particular choice of the origin,

$$\mathbf{r}_R = (0, 0, 0) \tag{13}$$

The torques of all three forces are

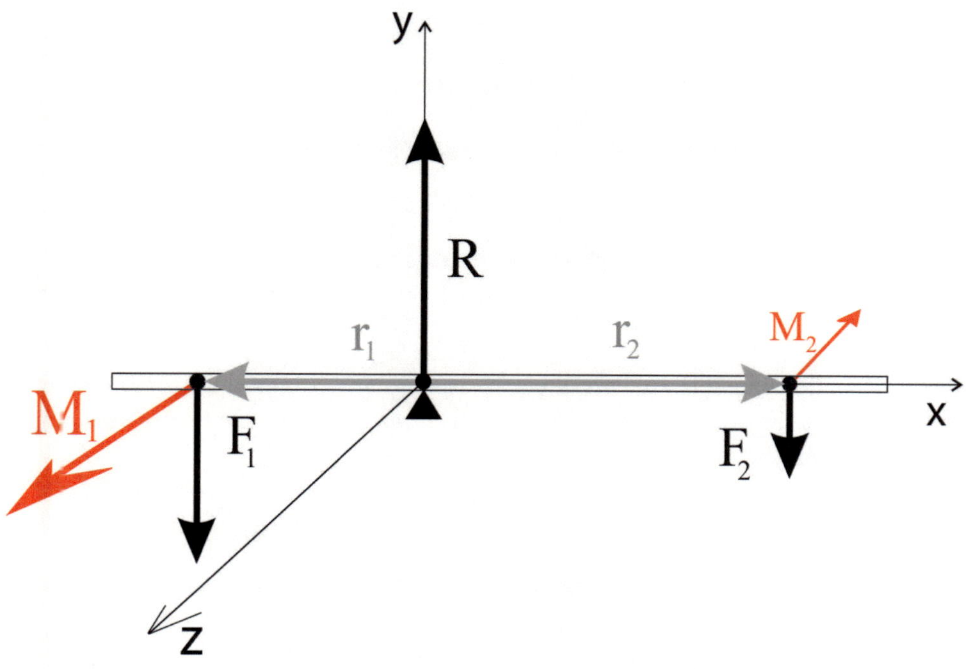

Figure 1. Scheme of a simple balance if the load forces act in the vertical direction.

$$\mathbf{M}_1 = \mathbf{r}_1 \times \mathbf{F}_1 = \begin{bmatrix} \mathbf{i} & \mathbf{j} & \mathbf{k} \\ -x_1 & 0 & 0 \\ 0 & -F_1 & 0 \end{bmatrix} = (0,\, 0,\, x_1 F_1) \tag{14}$$

$$\mathbf{M}_2 = \mathbf{r}_2 \times \mathbf{F}_2 = \begin{bmatrix} \mathbf{i} & \mathbf{j} & \mathbf{k} \\ x_2 & 0 & 0 \\ 0 & -F_2 & 0 \end{bmatrix} = (0,\, 0,\, -\, x_2 F_2) \tag{15}$$

$$\mathbf{M}_R = \mathbf{r}_R \times \mathbf{R} = \begin{bmatrix} \mathbf{i} & \mathbf{j} & \mathbf{k} \\ 0 & 0 & 0 \\ R_x & R_y & R_z \end{bmatrix} = (0,\, 0,\, 0) \tag{16}$$

In general, the equilibrium of forces is given by three equations for three components,

$$F_{1,x} + F_{2,x} + R_x = 0 \tag{17}$$

$$F_{1,y} + F_{2,y} + R_y = 0 \tag{18}$$

$$F_{1,z} + F_{2,z} + R_z = 0 \tag{19}$$

Following Eqs. (17)–(19), the components of the force R are

$$R_x = 0 \tag{20}$$

$$R_y = F_{1,y} + F_{2,y} \tag{21}$$

$$R_z = 0 \tag{22}$$

and the resultant force can be given as

$$\mathbf{R} = (0, F_1 + F_2, 0) \tag{23}$$

The equilibrium of torques is given by three equations for three components,

$$M_{1,x} + M_{2,x} + M_{R,x} = 0 \tag{24}$$

$$M_{1,y} + M_{2,y} + M_{R,y} = 0 \tag{25}$$

$$M_{1,z} + M_{2,z} + M_{R,z} = 0 \tag{26}$$

As the torque of the force **R** is equal to zero and also the components of the torques due to load forces in the x in y directions are equal to zero, there remains only one nontrivial equilibrium equation for torques,

$$M_{1,z} + M_{2,z} = 0 \tag{27}$$

Considering also the expressions (14) and (15), we obtain

$$x_1 F_1 - x_2 F_2 = 0 \tag{28}$$

and finally

http://dx.doi.org/10.5772/66753

$$\frac{F_1}{F_2} = \frac{x_2}{x_1} \tag{29}$$

2. A two-segment model for the resultant hip force in the one-legged stance

In a simple model of a one-legged stance (**Figure 2**), the body is divided into two segments: the loaded leg and the rest of the body (**Figure 2a**). The two segments are connected by the hip joint. **Figure 2b** presents an abstraction of the two segments (labeled I and II, respectively). For simplicity, the pelvis is taken to be leveled in the model. The sizes of the boxes correspond to approximate weight proportion of the two segments. Further, it is assumed that all the forces lie in the frontal plane of the body through the centers of both femoral heads (their components in the z direction are zero). The forces and momenta arms acting on the segment I are indicated in panels b and c. The hip is loaded at the medial side by the weight of the segment I (denoted as $\mathbf{W}_B - \mathbf{W}_L$), where $\mathbf{W}_B$ is the weight or the entire body and $\mathbf{W}_L$ is the weight of the loaded leg, and at the lateral side by a force of an effective muscle (denoted by $\mathbf{F}$), which pulls the segment toward the loaded leg. There are several muscles which are active in the one-legged stance, but in this simple model all of them are represented by one effective muscle with one origin at the crista iliaca and the other at the greater trochanter (**Figure 2c**). It is taken that the muscle force acts in the direction of the line connecting both origins, expressed by the inclination angle ϑ_F.

The model is based on equilibrium equations of forces and torques (Eqs. (1) and (2), respectively) acting on the segment I. Momentum arms of the weight of the segment I and of the

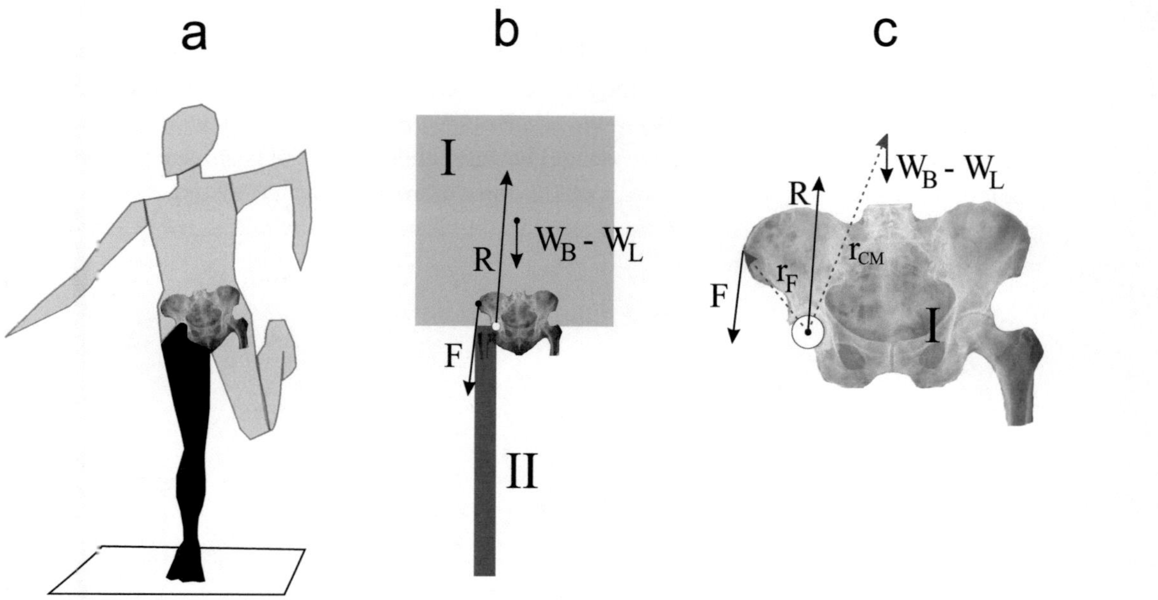

Figure 2. Scheme of a two-segment model of the one-legged stance. The body is divided into two segments: the loaded leg and the rest of the body (a). Abstraction of the two segments (labeled I and II, respectively) (b). Forces and their momentum arms (c).

effective muscle force can be determined from the geometry of the pelvis and proximal femur and the weight of the segment I can be determined from the body weight and an approximation that the leg weights about 1/7 of the entire body [1]. There are three unknown parameters in the model: the magnitude of the effective muscle force (F) and the magnitude and direction (inclination with respect to vertical) of the resultant hip force (R and ϑ_R, respectively).

2.1. A primitive model for resultant hip force

In the model (**Figures 3** and **4**), we have chosen the origin of the coordinate system at the center of the hip joint (that coincides with the center of the femoral head and the center of the acetabular shell). The loading forces are the weight of the segment I,

$$\mathbf{W}_{\mathrm{B}} - \mathbf{W}_{\mathrm{L}} = (0, -(W_{\mathrm{B}} - W_{\mathrm{L}}), 0), \tag{30}$$

with momentum arm $\mathbf{r}_{\mathrm{CM}}$,

$$\mathbf{r}_{\mathrm{CM}} = (x_{\mathrm{CM}}, y_{\mathrm{CM}}, 0) \tag{31}$$

and the force of the effective muscle, which lies in the frontal plane through centers of the femoral heads,

$$\mathbf{F} = (-F\cos\vartheta_F, -F\sin\vartheta_F, 0), \tag{32}$$

with momentum arm $\mathbf{r}_F$,

$$\mathbf{r}_F = (-x_F, y_F, 0). \tag{33}$$

The origin of the weight of the segment I is taken at the center of mass of the segment. It is approximated that this point lies in the sagittal plane of the body through the midline. Note that the components of the forces $\mathbf{W}_{\mathrm{B}} - \mathbf{W}_{\mathrm{L}}$ and $\mathbf{F}$ in the direction of the y-axis were taken to be negative, as these forces point downward and we have chosen that the positive direction of the y-axis is upward. Also, the component of the force $\mathbf{F}$ in the direction of the x-axis and the momentum arm of the effective muscle force in the direction of the x-axis are negative. The resultant hip force $\mathbf{R}$ is written as

$$\mathbf{R} = (R\sin\vartheta_R, R\cos\vartheta_R, 0). \tag{34}$$

The respective torques are

$$\mathbf{M}_{W_{\mathrm{B}}-W_{\mathrm{L}}} = \mathbf{r}_{\mathrm{CM}} \times (\mathbf{W}_{\mathrm{B}} - \mathbf{W}_{\mathrm{L}}) = \begin{bmatrix} \mathbf{i} & \mathbf{j} & \mathbf{k} \\ x_{\mathrm{CM}} & y_{\mathrm{CM}} & 0 \\ 0 & -(W_{\mathrm{B}} - W_{\mathrm{L}}) & 0 \end{bmatrix} = (0, 0, -x_{\mathrm{CM}}(W_{\mathrm{B}} - W_{\mathrm{L}})) \tag{35}$$

$$\mathbf{M}_F = \mathbf{r}_F \times \mathbf{F} = \begin{bmatrix} \mathbf{i} & \mathbf{j} & \mathbf{k} \\ -x_F & y_F & 0 \\ -F\cos\vartheta_F & -F\sin\vartheta_F & 0 \end{bmatrix} = (0, 0, x_F F\sin\vartheta_F + y_F F\cos\vartheta_F) \tag{36}$$

and

http://dx.doi.org/10.5772/66753

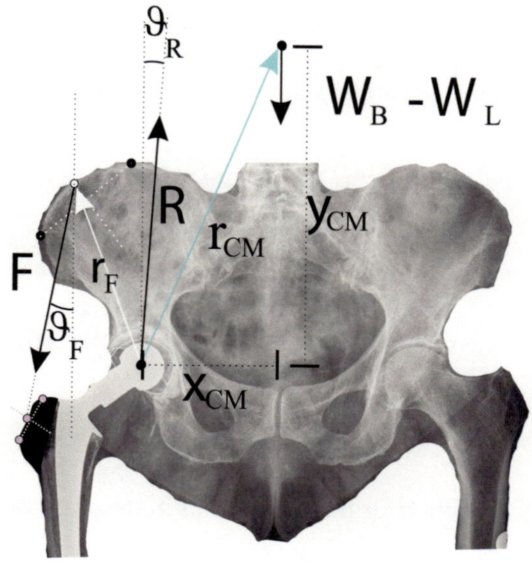

Figure 3. Scheme of forces and momentum arms in the primitive model subject to segment I.

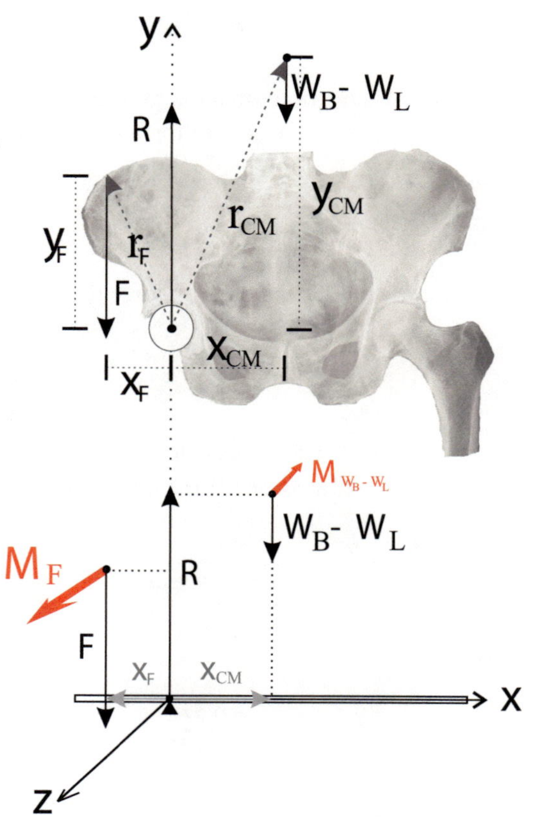

Figure 4. Scheme of a two-segment model of the one-legged stance.

$$\mathbf{M}_R = (0, 0, 0), \tag{37}$$

as the momentum arm of the resultant hip force is zero due to the choice of the origin of the coordinate system.

Following the above procedure, in particular Eq. (26), which describes equilibrium of torques, we obtain

$$-x_{\mathrm{CM}}(W_{\mathrm{B}} - W_{\mathrm{L}}) + F(x_F \sin \vartheta_F + y_F \cos \vartheta_F) = 0. \tag{38}$$

Rearranging the above equation yields for the unknown magnitude of the effective muscle force F,

$$F = \frac{x_{\mathrm{CM}}(W_{\mathrm{B}} - W_{\mathrm{L}})}{(x_F \cos \vartheta_F + y_F \sin \vartheta_F)}. \tag{39}$$

Following Eqs. (20)–(22), we obtain for the components in the direction of the x-axis

$$R \sin \vartheta_R = F \sin \vartheta_F \tag{40}$$

and in the direction of the y-axis

$$R \cos \vartheta_R = (W_{\mathrm{B}} - W_{\mathrm{L}}) + F \cos \vartheta_F. \tag{41}$$

Dividing Eq. (40) by Eq. (41) eliminates the unknown magnitude of the resultant hip force R and yields the expression for the inclination of the resultant force with respect to the vertical ϑ_R,

$$\tan \vartheta_R = \frac{\sin \vartheta_F}{\cos \vartheta_F + (W_{\mathrm{B}} - W_{\mathrm{L}})/F}. \tag{42}$$

By knowing F and ϑ_R, the magnitude of the resultant hip force R is then expressed from Eq. (40),

$$R = F\,\frac{\sin \vartheta_F}{\sin \vartheta_R}. \tag{43}$$

It is often convenient to present the results with respect to the body weight W_{B}. We also take into account that $W_{\mathrm{L}} = W_{\mathrm{B}}/7$ [2] to get the expression for the normalized effective muscle force

$$\frac{F}{W_{\mathrm{B}}} = \frac{6}{7}\frac{x_{\mathrm{CM}}}{(x_F \cos \vartheta_F + y_F \sin \vartheta_F)}, \tag{44}$$

the inclination of the resultant hip force

$$\tan \vartheta_R = \frac{\sin \vartheta_F}{\cos \vartheta_F + 6W_{\mathrm{B}}/7F}, \tag{45}$$

and the normalized resultant hip force

$$\frac{R}{W_{\rm B}} = \frac{6}{7}\left(1 + \frac{x_{\rm CM}}{x_F + y_F \tan \vartheta_F}\right). \tag{46}$$

In a special case when the effective muscle force points in the vertical direction, i.e., $\vartheta_F = 0$ (**Figure 4**), the expressions (44)–(46) simplify into

$$\frac{F}{W_{\rm B}} = \frac{6}{7}\frac{x_{\rm CM}}{x_F}, \tag{47}$$

$$\tan \vartheta_R = 0, \tag{48}$$

$$\frac{R}{W_{\rm B}} = \frac{6}{7}\left(1 + \frac{x_{\rm CM}}{x_F}\right). \tag{49}$$

Note that these expressions (Eqs. (47)–(49)) are the same as if obtained for a simple balance with the two loading forces

$$\mathbf{F}_1 = (0, -F, 0) \tag{50}$$

and

$$\mathbf{F}_2 = (0, -(W_{\rm B} - W_{\rm L}), 0) \tag{51}$$

and respective momentum arms

$$\mathbf{r}_F = (-x_F, 0, 0) \tag{52}$$

and

$$\mathbf{r}_{\rm CM} = (x_{\rm CM}, 0, 0). \tag{53}$$

Following Eqs. (29), (50), and (51), we obtain

$$\frac{F}{(W_{\rm B} - W_{\rm L})} = \frac{x_{\rm CM}}{x_F} \tag{54}$$

or (by taking into account that $W_{\rm L} = W_{\rm B}/7$)

$$\frac{F}{W_{\rm B}} = \frac{6}{7}\frac{x_{\rm CM}}{x_F}. \tag{55}$$

Following Eqs. (22), (50)–(51), and $W_{\rm L} = 6W_{\rm B}/7$, we obtain

$$R = F + \frac{6}{7}W_{\rm B}, \tag{56}$$

or, normalized

$$\frac{R}{W_B} = \frac{6}{7} + \frac{F}{W_B}. \tag{57}$$

Taking into account Eqs. (55) and (57) yields

$$\frac{R}{W_B} = \frac{6}{7}\left(1 + \frac{x_{CM}}{x_F}\right). \tag{58}$$

It can be seen that Eqs. (47) and (55) are identical. Likewise, Eqs. (49) and (58) are identical. Although the effective muscle attachment point on the iliac bone, the center of the femoral head, and the center of mass of the body segment I do not lie in the same horizontal plane, the model of simple balance derived for a weightless rigid bar with all forces originating in the same horizontal plane, gives the same solution, owing to a special case that the forces lie in the vertical direction only. It should however be kept in mind that this is a consequence of the simplifications used in the model of the one-legged stance and that in reality segment I has a characteristic shape that may impact the forces, which is not considered in the simple balance model. Some textbooks use a simple balance as an illustrative model to explain the principles of the effect of the muscle forces (the principles of different types of levers). It should be borne in mind that such approximations are valid only if all forces act in the same direction.

Figure 5 shows the dependence of the magnitude of the resultant hip force R on the ratio between parameters x_{CM} and x_F, for the primitive model with two different inclinations of the effective muscle force ($\vartheta_F = 20$ degrees, solid line, and $\vartheta_F = 10$ degrees, dotted line),

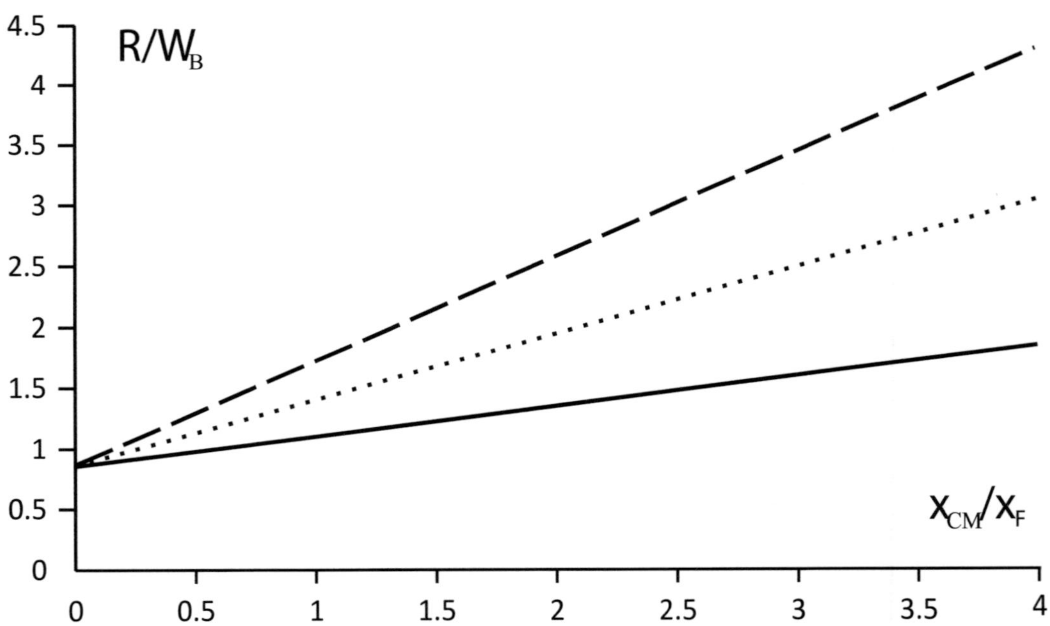

Figure 5. Dependence of the normalized resultant hip force R/W_B on the ratio between geometrical parameters x_{CM}/x_F for the primitive model (Eq. (46)) with two different inclinations of the effective muscle force ($\vartheta_F = 20$ degrees, solid line, and $\vartheta_F = 10$ degrees, dotted line), and for the simple balance model (Eq. (58)) (broken line). $y_F/x_F = 2$.

http://dx.doi.org/10.5772/66753

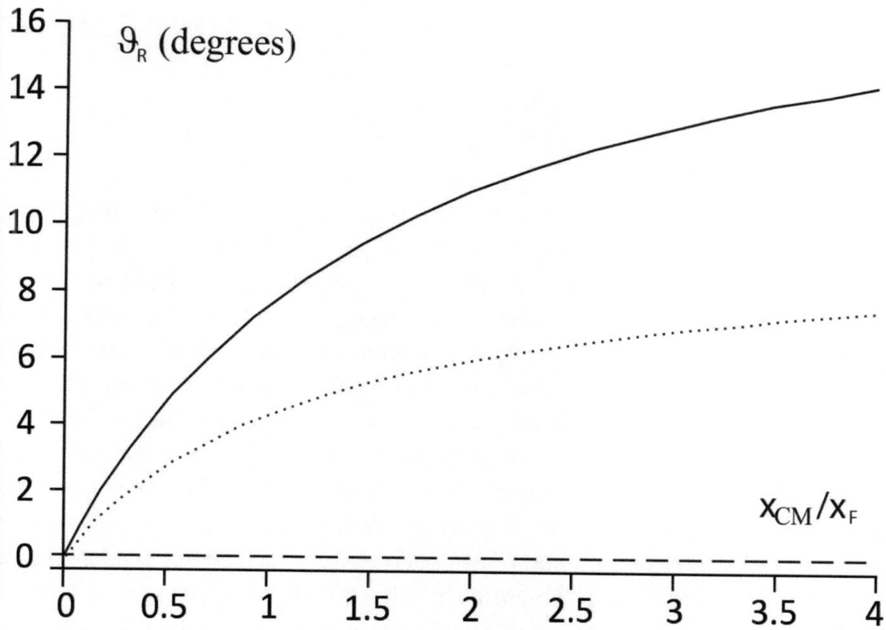

Figure 6. Dependence of the inclination of the resultant hip force with respect to vertical direction ϑ_R on the ratio between geometrical parameters x_{CM}/x_F for the primitive model (Eq. (45)) with two different inclinations of the effective muscle force ($\vartheta_F = 20$ degrees, solid line, and $\vartheta_F = 10$ degrees, dotted line), and for the simple balance model ($\vartheta_R = 0$, Eq. (48)) (broken line). $y_F/x_F = 2$.

and for the simple balance model (broken line). It can be seen that for larger x_{CM}/x_F and larger inclinations ϑ_F, the difference between the models becomes substantial. **Figure 6** shows the dependence of the inclination of the resultant hip force with respect to vertical direction ϑ_R on the ratio between parameters x_{CM} and x_F, for the primitive model with two different inclinations of the effective muscle force ($\vartheta_F = 20$ degrees, solid line, and $\vartheta_F = 10$ degrees, dotted line), and for the simple balance model (broken line). It can be seen that in the primitive model the inclination of the resultant hip force increases with increasing x_{CM}/x_F, the effect being more pronounced for larger inclination of the effective muscle force ϑ_F. In the simple balance model, the resultant hip force points in the direction of the y-axis (i.e., $\vartheta_R = 0$).

2.2. HIPSTRESS model for resultant hip force

The primitive model and the simple balance approximation consider only one muscle acting in a hip in the one-legged stance. Measurements however indicate that there are several muscles that are active in this body position. The static equilibrium requires that the resultant of all external forces acting on each segment is zero and that the resultant of all external torques acting on each segment is zero, therefore in a more realistic model, contributions of all active muscles should be taken into account. The equilibrium equation for forces acting on segment I is

$$\mathbf{W}_B - \mathbf{W}_L + \sum_i \mathbf{F}_i + \mathbf{R} = 0, \tag{59}$$

where index i runs over all muscles that are active in the one-legged stance. The equilibrium of torques is expressed by equation

$$\mathbf{r}_{\mathrm{CM}} \times (\mathbf{W}_{\mathrm{B}} - \mathbf{W}_{\mathrm{L}}) + \sum_{i} \mathbf{r}_i \times \mathbf{F}_i = 0, \tag{60}$$

where $\mathbf{r}_i$ is the momentum arms of the respective muscle forces and i runs over all the forces that are active in the one-legged stance. It was taken into account that the torque of the resultant hip force is zero since we have chosen the origin of the coordinate system in the center of the femoral head, that is, the origin of the resultant hip force. The HIPSTRESS model for resultant hip force takes into account nine effective muscles: gluteus minimus anterior, gluteus minimus middle, gluteus minimus posterior, gluteus medius anterior, gluteus medius middle, gluteus medius posterior, tensor fasciae latae, piriformis, and rectus femoris [2]. The geometry of the individual subject is taken into account by rescaling the coordinates of the reference muscle attachment points according to the geometry of the pelvis and proximal femur. However, if the standard anteroposterior radiogram is used to assess the geometrical parameters, only the coordinates in the directions of the x and y axes can be taken into account. The magnitude of the force of the i-th muscle is taken to be proportional to the muscle cross section area A_i and average tension in the muscle σ_i. Muscle forces are considered to act in straight lines between the muscle attachment points,

$$\mathbf{F}_i = A_i \sigma_i \frac{(\mathbf{r}_i - \mathbf{r'}_j)}{|\mathbf{r}_i - \mathbf{r'}_j|}, \tag{61}$$

where $\mathbf{r}_i$ is the coordinate of the origin of the i-th muscle on segment I and $\mathbf{r}'_i$ is the coordinate of the origin of the i-th muscle on segment II. Both coordinates are measured with respect to the center of the articular sphere (i.e., the center of the femoral head and the acteabular shell).

The forces and the torques have three dimensions, therefore the model consists of six equations (three for equilibrium of forces and three for equilibrium of torques). For known origin and insertion points of the muscles and known cross-section areas, the unknown quantities are the muscle tensions and three components of the resultant hip force R. Since there are 9 effective muscles and 3 components of the force R, there are 12 unknowns and 6 equations. To solve this problem, a simplification was introduced by dividing the muscles into three groups (anterior, middle, and posterior) with respect to the position. It was assumed that the muscles in the same group have the same tension. This reduced the number of unknowns to six as required for solution of the complex of six equations. The muscle origin and insertion points and the muscle cross-section were taken from Refs. [3] and [4], respectively. The geometry of the individual patient was taken into account by correction of muscle attachment points according to the geometrical parameters obtained from the standard anteroposterior radiograph, the distance from the center of the femoral head to the midline x_{CM}, the height of the pelvis H, the width of the pelvis C, and the position on the greater trochanter relative to the center of the femoral head x_{T} and y_{T} (**Figure 7**). Results obtained with the HIPSTRESS model for resultant hip force showed that the force lies almost in the frontal plane of the body through both femoral heads [1]. To further simplify the calculations it was assumed in most clinical studies

http://dx.doi.org/10.5772/66753

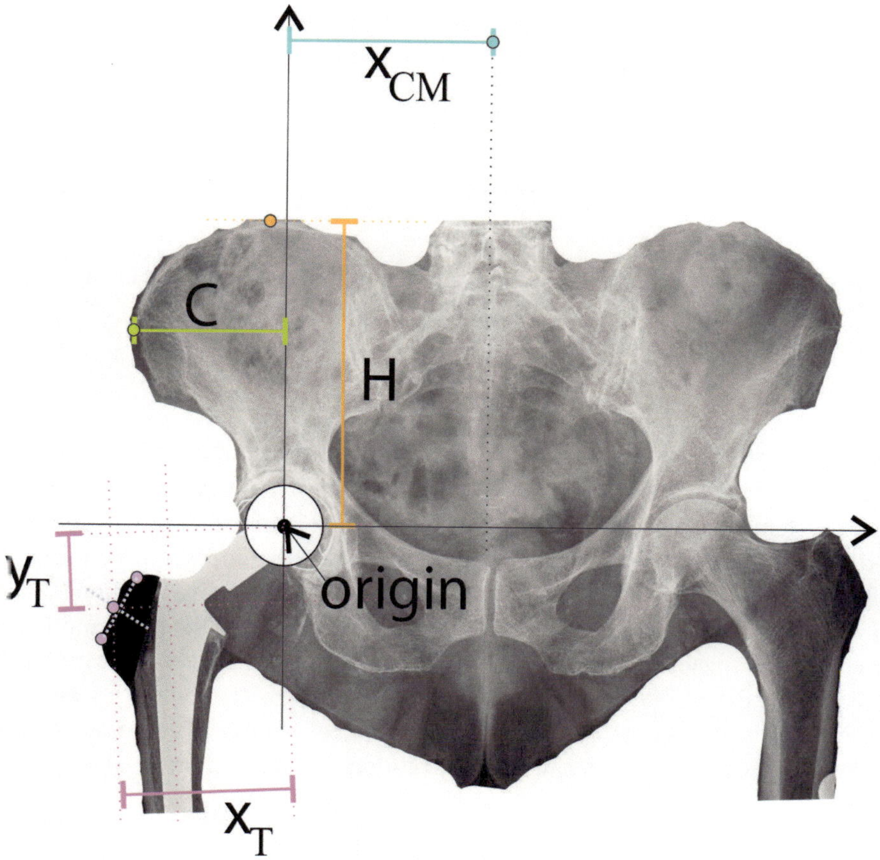

Figure 7. Geometrical parameters needed for determination of resultant hip force within the HIPSTRESS model.

using HIPSTRESS model that the force lies in the frontal plane and is, like in the primitive model, represented by its magnitude R and its inclination with respect to the vertical ϑ_R.

3. HIPSTRESS model for contact stress in the hip

Once we know what is the overall load **R** (the magnitude of the resultant hip force R and its inclination with respect to the vertical direction ϑ_R) that the hip must bear in order to keep the balance in the one-legged stance, it should also be clarified how this load is distributed over the load-bearing area. Namely, it is the local load that determines the development of cells. Therefore, we are interested in stresses connected to the load. The model HIPSTRESS for contact hip stress has previously been described in detail in Ref. [5]; therefore, only brief description will be given here. The readers who wish to understand the derivation of the equations are kindly asked to refer to the pointed literature.

We neglect all other stresses but the contact hip stress acting perpendicularly to the spherical articular surface, by assuming that the joint is well lubricated. A surface is imagined that is a part of a sphere with radius r, representing the hip joint. The contact hip stress p is connected to the resultant hip force,

$$\oint p \, \mathrm{d}\mathbf{A} = \mathbf{R}, \tag{62}$$

where $\mathbf{A}$ is the area element and the integration is performed over the load-bearing area of the articular surface.

It is assumed that stress is proportional to strain due to the squeezing of the cartilage between the femoral head and the acetabulum [6], which yields

$$p = p_0 \cos \gamma, \tag{63}$$

where p_0 is the stress at the stress pole and γ is the angle between the vector pointing from the origin of the coordinate system to the pole and the vector pointing from the origin of the coordinate system and the chosen point on the articular surface. The load-bearing area is bounded on the lateral side by the acetabular roof given in the radiogram by the center-edge angle of Wiberg ϑ_{CE} and on the medial side by the line where the cosine function (63) vanishes. Eq. (62) is represented by three equations for three components of the force and is subject to three unknown parameters of the model, that is, the position of the stress pole on the articular surface given by two angles Θ and Φ, and the value of stress at the pole p_0. The azimuthal angle of the pole is $\Phi = 0$ or π, as the resultant hip force in the one-legged stance lies in the frontal plane of the body. In order to get the solution for Θ, a nonlinear algebraic equation should be solved,

$$\tan(\vartheta_R + \Theta) = \frac{\cos^2(\vartheta_{\mathrm{CE}} - \Theta)}{\left(\frac{\pi}{2} + \vartheta_{\mathrm{CE}} - \Theta + \frac{1}{2}\sin(2(\vartheta_{\mathrm{CE}} - \Theta))\right)} \tag{64}$$

which simplifies into

$$\tan(x + y) = \frac{\cos^2(y - x)}{\left(\frac{\pi}{2} + (y - x) + \frac{1}{2}\sin(2(y - x))\right)} \tag{65}$$

by introducing the expressions

$$x = \Theta + \frac{1}{2}(\vartheta_R - \vartheta_{\mathrm{CE}}), \tag{66}$$

and

$$y = \frac{1}{2}(\vartheta_R + \vartheta_{\mathrm{CE}}). \tag{67}$$

As ϑ_R and ϑ_{CE} are the input parameters, and the unknown parameter is x, the solution of Eq. (64) is determined solely by the parameter y. The normalized value of stress at the pole is then expressed from

$$\frac{p_0 r^2}{R} = \frac{3}{2} \frac{\sin(y+x)}{\cos^2(y-x)}, \tag{68}$$

while its proper value can be calculated by multiplying the left side of Eq. (68) by R and dividing it by r^2. The polar angle is given by

$$\Theta = x - \frac{1}{2}(\vartheta_R - \vartheta_{CE}). \tag{69}$$

Figures 8 and **9** show the dependence of the polar angle and stress at the pole (Eqs. (69) and (68), respectively), on parameter y. Clinical studies that have validated the HIPSTRESS method have used the parameter peak stress on the weight-bearing area as the relevant quantity.

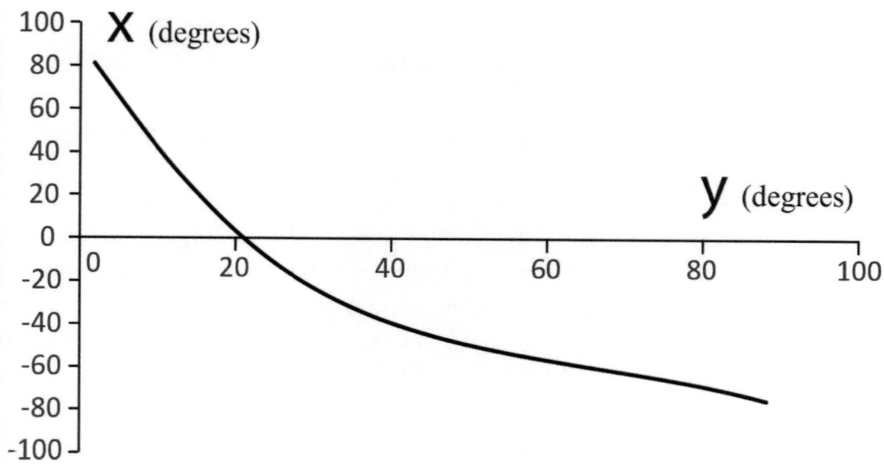

Figure 8. Dependence of the position of the pole Θ on parameter y.

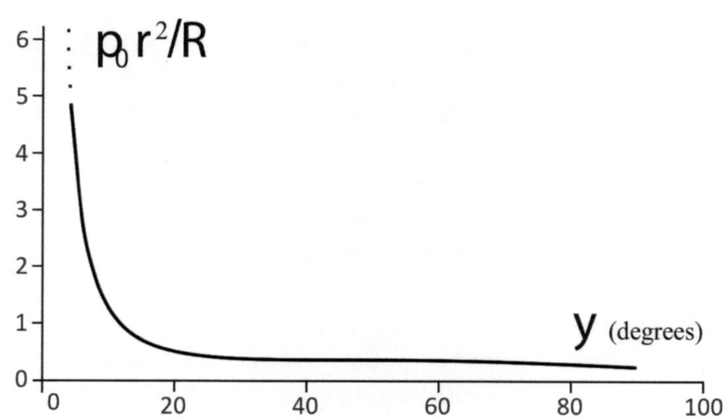

Figure 9. Dependence of the value of contact stress at the pole p_0 on parameter y.

Namely, the stress pole is an abstract point in which the respective spheres outlining the femoral head and the acetabulum most closely approach each other upon loading of the joint. The pole may therefore be located within the load-bearing area of the joint or outside it. In the first case, the peak stress is identical to the value of stress at the pole $p_{max} = p_0$, while in the second case, the peak stress is taken at the point on the load-bearing area that is closest to the stress pole. If this takes place at the acetabular rim, the peak stress is calculated according to the expression $p_{max} = p_0 \cos(\vartheta_{CE} - \Theta)$ [5]. It was shown that biomechanical parameters calculated with HIPSTRESS models for resultant hip force and contact hip stress were useful in explaining early osteoarthritis in dysplastic hips [7], hips with primary osteoarthritis, hips subject to avascular necrosis of the femoral head [5], hips that were in childhood subject to the Perthes disease [8], effect of different osteotomies [9–12], and the direction and volumetric wear of total hip endoprosthesis [13]. Evidently, the models include the relevant parameters of the individual hip to have a predictive value.

4. Comparison of the primitive model and the HIPSTRESS model

The primitive model and the HIPSTRESS model both use the same characteristic points on the iliac bone and on the greater trochanter (i.e., the highest and the most lateral points). In both models, the center-edge angle and the radius of the articular surface (i.e., the radius of the femoral head) is needed to calculate stress distribution. Both models consider the center of mass and the corresponding momentum arm. There are however differences in parameters for the resultant hip force. The HIPSTRESS model includes more parameters (H, C, x_{CM}, x_T, and y_T) than the primitive model (x_{CM}, x_F, and ϑ_F) to characterize geometry of the individual hip and pelvis. The parameters of HIPSTRESS (but not the primitive model) enable consideration of the inclination of the femoral neck.

For illustration we calculate the biomechanical parameters by using both models and also the simple balance approximation. **Figure 10** shows the measured geometrical parameters for the primitive model and **Figure 11** shows the measured parameters for the HIPSTRESS model.

To determine the magnitude and the inclination of the resultant hip force (R and ϑ_R, respectively) in the primitive model, we use the measured parameters and Eqs. (44)–(46), while in the simple balance approximation, with $\vartheta_R = 0$, R is obtained by using Eq. (58). To estimate R and ϑ_R in the HIPSTRESS model, we used the nomograms as described in [1]. The results of all three models are depicted in **Table 1**. It can be seen that for the chosen hip and pelvis, the magnitude of the resultant hip force in the primitive model and in the HIPSTRESS model differ by only 9%, while in the simple balance approximation the result deviates by about 40%. The inclination of the resultant hip force ϑ_R is by definition zero in the simple balance approximation, but it is also small in the primitive model and in the HIPSTRESS model. By using these results we can estimate the parameter y in all three models. Knowing y, we estimate also parameter x in all three models by using **Figure 10**. Parameter x is needed to calculate the position of the pole Θ by using Eq. (69). Finally, the value of stress at the pole is obtained by using the respective values of y and **Figure 9**. The inset of the figure with the values corresponding to all three models is shown in **Figure 12**.

http://dx.doi.org/10.5772/66753

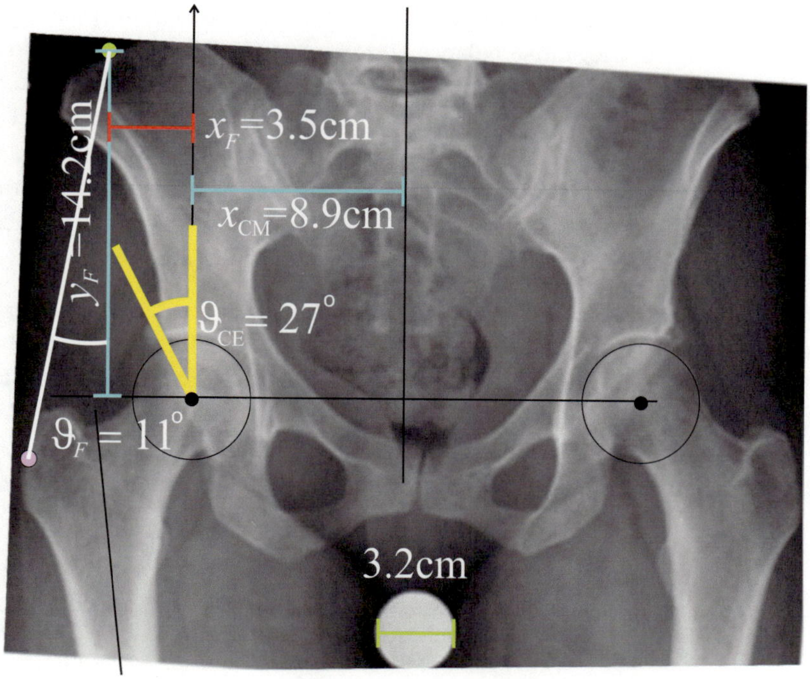

Figure 10. Geometrical parameters needed for the determination of the resultant hip force within the primitive model.

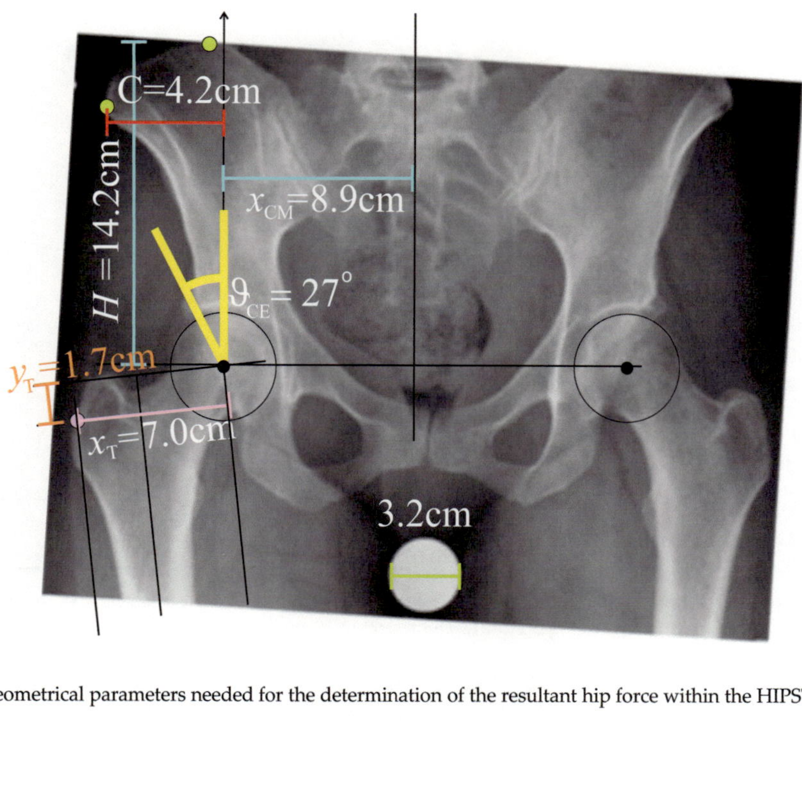

Figure 11. Geometrical parameters needed for the determination of the resultant hip force within the HIPSTRESS model.

It can be seen that in the primitive model and in the HIPSTRESS model the pole lies within the load-bearing area while in the simple balance approximation it falls outside the load-bearing area (**Table 1**). The HIPSTRESS model in this case yields the lowest stress. Note that in the simple balance approximation the hip would according to the criteria of the HIPSTRESS [14, 15] be considered as dysplastic since it exhibits rapidly decreasing stress at the lateral acetabular rim. However, the center-edge angle is 27° which is considered as a healthy hip. The simple balance model overestimates hip stress and is in most cases not suitable to give quantitative result regarding biomechanical parameters of the hip and pelvis.

The example that we have shown corresponds to a normal hip geometry. Also, the values of peak stress that were obtained by the primitive model and the HIPSTRESS model are within the values corresponding to hips that would remain without clinical problems up to about 85 years of age [16]. In this case, the primitive model proved successful in estimating biomechanical parameters. However, to see whether it has a predictive value, it should be validated by clinical studies. The advantage of the primitive model is that it is simpler and does not need

Parameter	SBA	Primitive	HIPSTRESS
r (cm)	2.47	2.47	2.47
ϑ_{CE} (degrees)	27	27	27
x_{CM} (cm)	8.9	8.9	8.9
x_F (cm)	3.5	3.5	
y_F (cm)	14.2	14.2	
ϑ_F (degrees)	0	11	
C (cm)			4.2
H (cm)			14.6
x_T (cm)			7.0
y_T (cm)			1.7
R/W_B	3.2	2.2	2.4
ϑ_R (degrees)	0	7	12
y	13.3	17	20
x	27	12	2
p_0/W_B (m^{-2})	4693	2693	2172
p_{max}/W_B (m^{-2})	4572	2693	2172
Θ(degrees)	40	22	10

SBA, simple balance approximation.

Table 1. Geometrical and biomechanical parameters for a hip with total hip endoprothesis as determined by simple balance approximation, primitive model and HIPSTRESS model of a one leged stance.

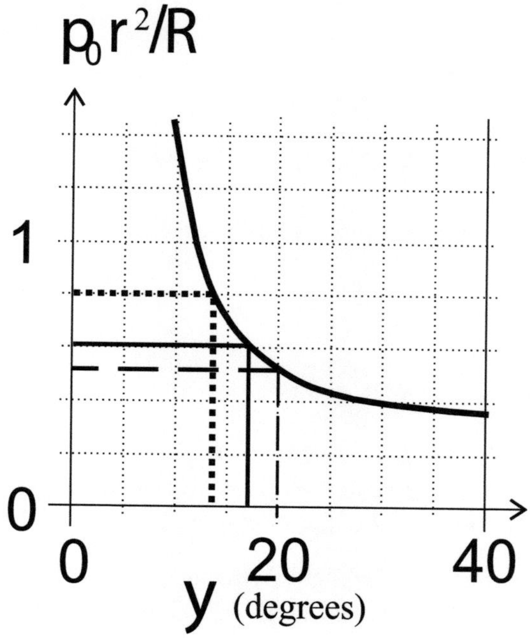

Figure 12. Estimation of the value of p_0 for the primitive model (solid lines), simple balance approximation (dotted lines), and HIPSTRESS model (broken lines).

special software. Determination of the resultant hip force with the primitive model is scale independent which is an advantage over the HIPSTRESS model. Namely, the HIPSTRESS model uses three-dimensional coordinates of the muscle attachment points of a reference hip and pelvis but only the x and y coordinates are rescaled according to the hip considered, while the z coordinates of the reference hip remain in the model. Therefore, the HIPSTRESS model for the resultant hip force is biased by the artifact that it depends on the size of the hip.

We have used standard anteroposterior radiograms to measure geometrical parameters. Imaging with magnetic resonance has recently improved to enable determination of three-dimensional positions of muscle attachment points for the needs of the HIPSTRESS method, but has not yet been used for the determination of biomechanical parameters by this method. This would be a major improvement over using radiograms, as the direct data on the muscle attachment points could be used and there would be no need for rescaling of the reference geometry. In considering the three-dimensional data the primitive model could not do justice to the system as its assumptions are bounded to the simplification to two dimensions. However, the primitive model (but not the simple balance approximation) merits to minimal standards to be used for understanding of the principles of the equilibrium of forces and torques in the one-legged stance, and can in certain cases (such as the one shown here) also yield a valid quantitative estimation of the biomechanical parameters.

Author details

Veronika Kralj-Iglič

Address all correspondence to: veronika.kralj-iglic@fe.uni-lj.si

Laboratory of Clinical Biophysics, Faculty of Health Sciences, University of Ljubljana, Ljubljana, Slovenia

References

[1] Kralj-Iglic V (2015). Validation of mechanical hypothesis of hip arthritis development by HIPSTRESS method. Osteoarthritis - Progress in Basic Research and Treatment, Chen Q (Ed.), InTech, Rijeka, Croatia, DOI: 10.5772/59976.

[2] Iglic A, Srakar F, Antolic V, Kralj-Iglic V, Batagelj V (1990). Mathematical analysis of Chiari osteotomy. *Acta Orthop Iugosl*, 20, 35–39.

[3] Dostal WF, Andrews JG (1981). A three-dimensional biomechanical model of the hip musculature. *J Biomech*, 14, 803–812.

[4] Johnston RC, Brand RA, Crowninshield RD (1979). Reconstruction of the hip. *J Bone Joint Surg*, 61A, 639–652.

[5] Kralj-Iglic V, Dolinar D, Ivanovski M, List I, Daniel M (2012). Role of biomechanical parameters in hip osteoarthritis and avascular necrosis of femoral head. Applied Biological Engineering - Principles and Practice, Naik GR (Ed.), InTech, Rijeka, Croatia, DOI: 10.5772/30159.

[6] Brinckmann P, Frobin W, Hierholzer E (1981). Stress on the articular surface of the hip joint in healthy adults and persons with idiopathic osteoarthrosis of the hip joint. *J Biomech*, 14, 149–156, ISSN 0044-3220.

[7] Mavcic B, Pompe B, Antolic V, Daniel M, Iglic A, Kralj-Iglic V (2002). Mathematical estimation of stress distribution in normal and dysplastic human hips. *J Orthop Res*, 20, 1025–1030.

[8] Kocjancic B, Molicnik A, Antolic V, Mavcic B, Kralj-Iglic V, Vengust R (2014). Unfavorable hip stress distribution after Legg-Calve-Perthes syndrome: a 25-year follow-up of 135 hips. *J Orthop Res*, 32, 8–16.

[9] Herman S, Jaklic A, Herman S, Iglic A, Kralj-Iglic V (2002). Hip stress reduction after Chiari osteotomy. *Med Biol Eng Comput*, 40, 369–375.

[10] Dolinar D, Antolič V, Herman S, Iglic A, Kralj-Iglic V, Pavlovcic V (2003). Influence of contact hip stress on the outcome of surgical treatment of hips affected by avascular necrosis. *Arch Orthop Trauma Surg*, 123, 509–513, ISSN 0936-8051

[11] Kralj M, Mavcic B, Antolic V, Iglic A, Kralj-Iglic V (2005). The Bernese periacetabular osteotomy: clinical, radiographic and biomechanical 7-15 year follow-up in 26 hips. *Acta Orthop*, 76, 833–840, ISSN 1745-3674

[12] Vukasinovic Z, Spasovski D, Kralj-Iglic V, Marinkovic-Eric J, Seslija I, Zivkovic Z, Spasovski V (2013). Impact of triple pelvic osteotomy on contact stress pressure distribution in the hip joint. *Intl Orthopaed*, 37(1), 95–98. doi:10.1007/s00264-012-1727-y.

[13] Rijavec B, Kosak R, Daniel M, Kralj-Iglic V, Dolinar D (2014). Effect of cup inclination on predicted stress-induced volumetric wear in total hip replacement. *Comput Meth Biomech Biomed Eng*, 18(13), 1468–73.

[14] Pompe B, Antolic V, Mavcic B, Iglic A, Kralj-Iglic V (2007). Hip joint contact stress as an additional parameter for determining hip dysplasia in ad ults: comparison with Severins classification. *Med Sci Monit*, 13, CR215–219.

[15] Pompe B, Daniel M, Sochor M, Vengust R, Kralj-Iglic V, Iglic A (2003). Gradient of contact stress in normal and dysplastic human hips. *Medical Eng Phys*, 25, 379–385, ISSN 1350-4533

[16] Mavcic B, Slivnik T, Antolic V, Iglic A, Kralj-Iglic V (2004). High contact hip stress is related to the development of hip pathology with increasing age. *Clin Biomech*, 19(9), 939–943. doi: 10.1016/j.clinbiomech.2004.06.003

Chapter 3

Developmental Dysplasia of the Hip in Childhood – Etiology, Diagnostics and Conservative Treatment

Ismet Gavrankapetanović and Adnan Papović

Additional information is available at the end of the chapter

http://dx.doi.org/10.5772/67481

Abstract

Since developmental dysplasia of the hip (DDH) represents one of the most common congenital deformations of the musculoskeletal system and the most common deformation of the hip joint, the aim is to emphasize the importance of early recognition and diagnosis of DDH as well as comprehensive screening among newborns. DDH represents a dynamic process that results in the action of a number of exogenous and endogenous factors, physiological and mechanical, exerted to the mother and to the child during pregnancy and after delivery. Summary of all current knowledge about the origin of this deformity suggests that the most important factors in the development are hard abdominal muscles and uterine muscles, as limiting factors for fetal movement, which prevents its physiological turn, and reinforces the pelvic presentation of the fetus in uterus. Considering the fact that developmental dysplasia of the hip demands multidisciplinary approach and cooperation among gynecologists, neonatologists, pediatricians, radiologists, and orthopedic surgeons, the goal of this chapter is to make a consensus about early conservative treatment among clinicians, time of commencement, and its efficacy.

Keywords: developmental dysplasia of the hip, conservative treatment, early commencement, hip ultrasonography, Risser traction, cast shorts

1. Introduction

Developmental dysplasia of the hip (DDH[1]) represents the most common congenital deformation of the musculoskeletal system, ahead of the congenital talipes equinovarus and torticollis. Statistical data of the frequency of occurrence of this deformity in Bosnia and Herzegovina states that one of the forms of developmental dysplasia of the hip occurs in 3–5% of all births.

The data is probably not definitive and variable, and certainly depends on geographical distribution, the degree of health care education, the organization of the health care system and many other factors. Developmental dysplasia of the hip more often occurs in some countries and regions. In Bosnia and Herzegovina, the frequency rate of one of the forms of developmental dysplasia of the hip is the largest in the whole of Europe (Sweden 1.7, Bosnia and Herzegovina 75 on 1000 newborns). To what extent will they be recorded depends on the other two factors. Probably, only in economically developed countries, it is possible to implement an adequate screening method, thus adequately examine all newborn children, in order to identify hip deformities and start the treatment in the most appropriate period of time. In countries where the health care system is still in development, including Bosnia and Herzegovina, medical attention to possible occurrence of some form of developmental dysplasia of the hip is mainly directed toward the high risk groups. The great importance was previously given to the genetic nature of the DDH has been generally reduced. The reason lies in the fact that there are a large number of children with healthy hip genetically marked for DDH, but also a large number of children with malformed hips without a positive family history. The pelvic presentation of the fetus at birth, for most of the authors is considered the group at greatest risk.

DDH can be associated with other anomalies of the musculoskeletal system, first of all with torticollis, and foot deformities called *pes metatarsus congenitus varus*. The gender distribution shows that DDH occurs more often in female children than in male children with ratio of 4:1. According to some authors, the mildest form of this deformity is equally present in both sexes, while the more severe forms are more often presented in female children, with the left hip more often affected than the right, noting that serious forms are twice more frequent than most lenient.

For a long period, wandering in its search for names for all degrees of congenital deformities of the hip, speaks enough about the complexity of the pathoanatomical changes on the deformed hip. As the mechanism of DDH still remains unclear, for our purposes we will mainly use the knowledge gathered up to now. Thus, DDH represents a dynamic process that results in the action of a number of exogenous and endogenous factors, physiological and mechanical, exerted to the mother and to the child during pregnancy and after delivery. Therefore, we are talking about a multifactorial etiology of DDH. As a predisposing factor in the course of the development of deformity is a loose joint capsule. The mechanism of hip dislocation in children is consisted in the fact that in fetal pelvic presentation, hips are in maximal flexion and knees in maximal extension. The muscles of the posterior aspect of the upper leg cause an increased pressure of the proximal part of the femur on the articular capsule and the head gradually slipping from the acetabulum. Further progression of the deformity flow is accelerated in the postnatal period with traditional practices of diapering a child (with a cloth), present in our country, with maximum outstretched legs. The reason is that a newborn baby has a congenital flexion contracture of 15° caused by the intrauterine fetal position. Forced extension with shortened *m. iliopsoas* (this muscle is given a big role in the formation of DDH), leading formation of one of the forms of this deformity. The pathoanatomical substrate shows different degrees of deformity of joint elements. The head of the femur is due to cartilage material commonly deformed, and a degree of deformity varies from case to case. It is most commonly deformed from its back side, although cases are known when it is a normal, spherical shape [1].

http://dx.doi.org/10.5772/67481

2. Developmental dysplasia of the hip

Deformities of the femoral neck also depend on the moment of recognition of DDH, ranging from shortened neck with a slight ante version, and normal CD angle, to a significant shortening of the neck and greater ante version with a significant increase in CD angle. Analog to removal of the femoral head from the bottom of the acetabulum, comes the prolonging and thickening of *ligamentum teres capitis*. Depending on the degree of DDH, new changes are reflected on the acetabulum as well. In the mildest form of deformity, the acetabulum is shallow, the roof is steep, and the smallest part covers the head of the femur. When it comes to more severe deformities, subluxation or dislocations, acetabulum as a natural cavity, since empty, now tends to close, doing it by pulvinar and hypertrophic *ligamentum teres capitis*. The oval shape of a healthy acetabulum becomes triangular. Limbus in dysplastic hips becomes rounded, while in the luxated hips it is inverted and does not allow the luxated head of the femur bone to reposition in the acetabulum. The joint capsule is loose in each case and stretched. Because of the tendency of the femoral head to travel proximally, the joint capsule gets stretched from the front, and narrowed in the space between the femoral head and the acetabulum, due to effects of a hypertrophic and shortened *m. iliopsoas*. It advances along the outside of the iliac bone and gets a look of an 'hourglass.' This narrowing, the so called isthmus, with an inverted limbus creates an insurmountable obstacle with the luxated head of the femur to its repositioning. All of these changes in the joint elements do not pass the muscles around them. This primarily refers to adductor muscles and *m. iliopsoas*, which is shortened and hypertrophied.

All mentioned so far about developmental dysplasia of the hip (DDH) speaks to the fact that this is a dynamic process; thus, we are more assured in the knowledge that the recently adopted name can completely suppress the previously rigid 'congenital hip dislocation.' For this reason, even quite simple classification into three basic levels of deformity of the hip cannot meet our needs. For practical reasons, we will use the classification depending on the age of the child, because of the clinical presentation, diagnosis, and treatment options

For the *newborn of 3 months old*, because of the characteristic clinical features, great possibilities of using ultrasound diagnostics, and limited possibility of using X-rays, following classification is used:

1. Loose hip: joint elements are positioned in satisfactory relation and we are not able to do a manual dislocation, but there is a significant stretching of soft tissues and ligaments, and the separation of the femoral head from the acetabulum.

2. Luxable hip: such hip where we can do a manual dislocation, joint elements are in a satisfactory relationship, but slack joint capsule and ligaments allow luxation, where the head of the femur spontaneously reduces when the pressure of the hand ceases.

3. Luxated hip: the head of the femur is out of the acetabulum, and repositioning is performed with Ortolani maneuver.

For *children older than 3 months,* following classification is used:

1. Displastic hip: joint bodies are in a satisfactory relationship, but acetabulum is shallow with a steep roof.
2. Subluxated hip: the head of the femur is only in partial contact with the outer part of the acetabulum.
3. Luxated hip: the head of the femur is located outside the acetabulum in the soft tissues.

2.1. Incidence

In about 60% of patients the left hip is affected, about 20% both, and the remaining 20% patients the right hip is affected. Although the cause of disease is found to be multifactorial, still there are certain conditions that can be extracted, characteristics of medical history and risks that show a significant correlation with the incidence of DDH:

1. ligament hyperlaxity;
2. increased femoral antetorsion;
3. decreased acetabular antetorsion;
4. intrauterine malposition;
5. positive family history;
6. firstborn;
7. sectio cesarea;
8. oligohydramnion;
9. gemini and multiple pregnancy;
10. female gender; and
11. more frequent reporting with following orthopedic diseases: metatarsus varus, pes calcaneovalgus, torticollis, plagiocephalia, extensor knee contracture.

2.2. Clinical presentation

Clinical examination of the newborn should comply with all instructions relating to the pediatric examination of the child, which means that the child should be examined in a warm room, the table covered with clean and dry diaper cloth, provided only for child examination. Access to child should be in accordance to its behavior, and examination should be carried out gently, but with firm movements. The child lies on its back; an examination should begin with maximum, but not forced extension of the hip and knee, pulling the foot while pushing the knees with your thumb. In doing so, first pay attention to the length of the limb, because shortening speaks for dislocations to abbreviated side. Further attention

http://dx.doi.org/10.5772/67481

should focus on the presence of gluteofemoral and gluteogenital skin creases, as well as folds in the thigh.

The asymmetry of the folds, even if it does not represent the 'Bade diagnostic sign' especially in the newborn, still speaks in favor of the possible occurrence of DDH. What follows in the examination is flexion of the hip and knee while closely observing the knees which are in healthy children in the same level, and in children with affected side causes the lowering of knee level. The examiner now places hands on the knees applying slight pressure in the axial direction. On the side of possible dislocation elastic hip plunging can be observed. Further examination is continued with characteristic posture of orthopedic hip examination in children. Palm of the examiner is placed on knees, thumb on the medial side of the thigh, and the other fingers on the lateral side where the tip of the middle finger is placed on the great trochanter. Hips of the child are flexed in 90°. We perform flexion and extension of the hip, with attention to the trochanter. 'The walking' of trochanter is a sign of its dislocation or luxation, sometimes with the phenomenon of squeaking of the femoral head against the hip, therefore we talk about the positive Hoffa's sign. Hips are further abducted. In newborns there is an abductor contracture of 45°, and in infants of 60°. Greater values of this abductor contracture are signs of either some form of DDH or hypertonus of the adductor muscles and *m. iliopsoas*.

The values of the abduction of more than 90°, or hyperabduction on the other hand, are a sure diagnostic sign of dislocation.

Characteristic positive signs in the diagnosis of DDH represent 'skipping signs,' Ortolani sign of reposition and Palmen luxation sign. The first is carried out in a manner that in the position of abducted hips, examiner's middle finger is putting a pressure on the femur head and with that pressure it is pushed forward. Dislocated head is pushed over the back edge of the acetabulum, where the examiner can feel the distinctive phenomenon of 'skipping' or 'clicking.' Palmen luxation leap is caused by the applied pressure on the knee in the axial direction with hips in adduction position.

In luxable hips one can feel the characteristic 'overriding phenomenon,' which is caused by the femur head crossing over the dysplastic acetabulum.

After removal of the pressure on the knee there is a spontaneous repositioning. This completes the orthopedic hips examination in children (**Figure 1**). It is important to note that certain diagnostic signs hold greater importance depending on the age of the child, so we distinguish clinical examination of newborns and infants. The value of Ortolani and Palmen sign decreases as child grows older. The reason for this lies in secondary changes in the bones and soft tissues in terms of shortening and hypertrophy of adductor muscles and *m. iliopsoas*. On the other hand, importance of asymmetric skin folds' findings of gluteofemoral and genitofemoral region increases. At the same time there can be noted limited abduction, which is an important diagnostic sign for DDH in older children. For older children, at walking age, there is a characteristic-waddling gait on luxated side, which indicates the positive Trendelburg sign. Compensatory, in order to maintain balance, the child leans the upper body to the burdened party, which is a positive sign of Duchenne. When mutual dislocations are a finding, there can be noted distinctive 'duck walk,' with increased lumbar lordosis. Further verification of the possible positive clinical diagnostic signs need to be done by ultrasound and X-ray diagnostics.

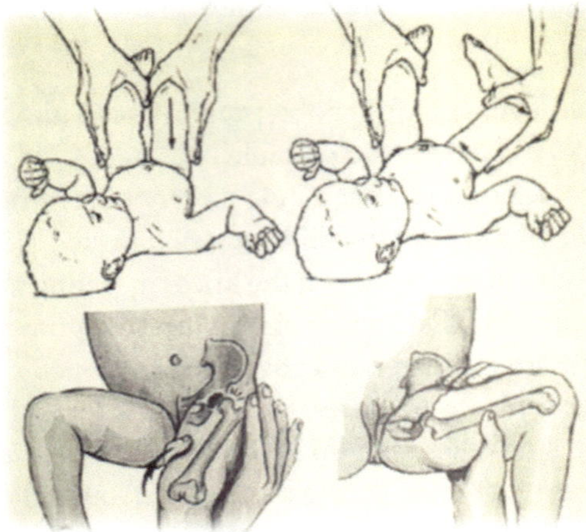

Figure 1. Two left images show Palmen test (provoked luxation), and two right images show Ortolani test (reposition of the luxated hip).

2.3. Diagnosis

According to all authors, ultrasound waves of 7.5 MHz frequency are completely harmless, which entails the conclusion that the ultrasound diagnosis of the hip disease in children is the most appropriate and harmless diagnostic way (**Figure 2**).

The method is simple and can be repeated. Among diagnostic methods, it is the preferred one, because it can give a diagnosis in the first days of life and refer us to the most appropriate treatment.

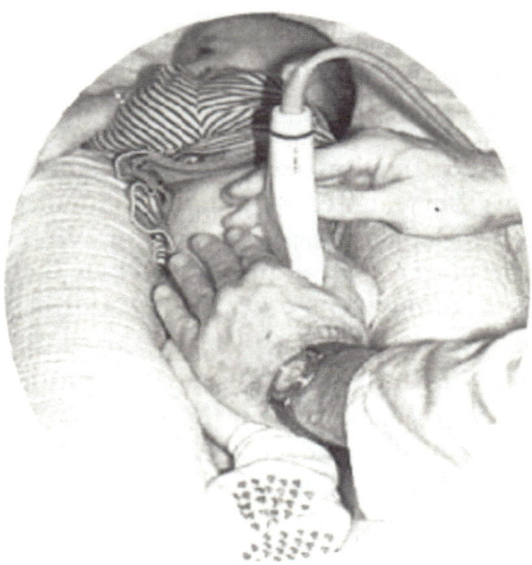

Figure 2. Child hip examination ultrasound.

http://dx.doi.org/10.5772/67481

Radiographic diagnostics, which was mainly used in our country, in addition to its proven harmful effects, is very difficult and misleading. The first months of life are crucial, for setting up possible diagnosis as well, because according to the data, the healing rate in open hip anomalies in the first month is 100%, yet already in the fourth month of life this percentage falls to 60%. This in itself speaks about the benefits of ultrasound diagnostics. Here we note the importance of quality and detailed ultrasound examination and extremely patient clinician, because even a small mistake, a small loss of patience or noncompliance of procedure can result in serious diagnostic failures with unforeseeable consequences.

We suggest an ultrasound hip screening of every baby up to 4 months of age without a specific indication. Of course that the positive family history, hormonal maintained pregnancy, oligohydramnios, pelvic presentation and caesarean section, indicate grounds for a pediatrician to send a child to children's orthopaedist as soon as possible.

An examination is performed in the lateral decubitus. Stability assessment is carried out through the assessments of the femur epiphysis and acetabulum, and by determining the angular parameters of bone and cartilage edge of the acetabulum on the sonogram (**Figure 3**).

Rather informatively, in short we list the Graphs infant hip classification based on ultrasound examination:

Type I: Fits to mature newborn hip, bone formation of acetabulum is good, but part of the acetabular cartilage supplements the bony part, thus the acetabular roof is completed.

Type II: Bone formation is not satisfactory, the cartilage roof is extended. Here we say that there is a delay in bone development.

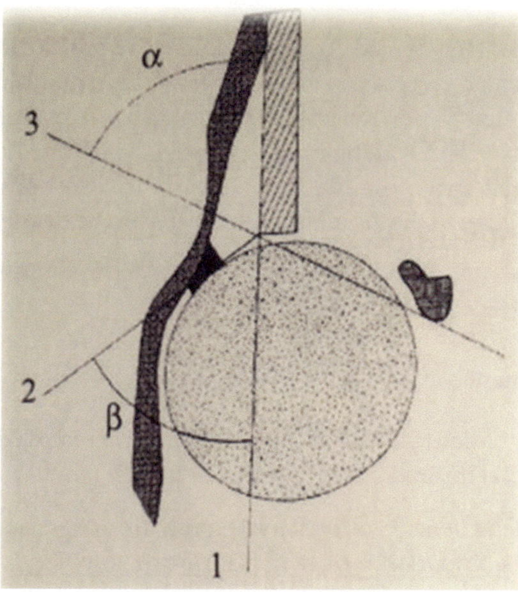

Figure 3. Schematic draws of diagnosis, using ultrasound with alpha and beta angles, based on marked lines 1, 2, and 3.

Type III: Cartilage part of the acetabular roof is deformed and pushed in craniolateral direction.

Type IV: Femoral head is luxated in dorsocranial direction. The entrance to the acetabulum is closed [2].

In this section, we will talk about subtypes and the morphometric ultrasonic hip balance change with reference lines, points, and angles.

Radiological diagnostic, after clinical and ultrasound examination leads to a definitive diagnosis of DDH. This type of examination is used only after 3 months of age. The reason lies in the fact that in the first 3 months, the reference bone structures are insufficiently developed, thus the recorded image is not suitable for interpretation. Technically, the imaging is done in the AP position, the child lies on its back with his feet together, with a mild hip and knee flexion of 30° in order to avoid the impact of the lumbar lordosis. Central rays are directed to the pubic symphysis, while protecting the gonads of a child, especially of male gender.

With interpretation, in order to avoid subjectivity, we use the extra lines that pave the X-ray of the pelvis with the hips:

1. Hilgenreiner line or Y line passing through Y crack.
2. Ombredann-Parkinson line perpendicularly cuts prior line and passes through the lateral edge of acetabulum.
3. Acetabular line passes along the edge of the roof of acetabulum.
4. Shenton-Menard line or cervical-obturatorious arc in healthy individuals it represents an unbroken line passing along the medial edge of the femur and continuing to the upper edge of obturator opening.

Squares incurred by crossing the first two lines define the position of the femoral head. In healthy hips, the head is placed regularly in the lower medial square, in subluxated hips in the lower lateral, and in luxated hips in the upper lateral square. Acetabular index represents the angle formed by Y cartilage and acetabular line crossing. After birth, acetabular index should not exceed 30°, and in the third year 20°. In infants, the value of acetabular index of 24° or more with the rounded edge of the acetabulum speaks in favor of a dysplastic hip (**Figure 4**).

In addition to the above mentioned diagnostic methods, arthrography, CT scan of the hip, and MRI are also used, but very rarely [3, 4].

2.4. Conservative treatment

Here we perform a strict division to the conservative treatment, which is possible in the first months of a child's life, and surgical treatment which we prefer in later months of child development.

We strongly emphasize the benefits of preventive measures, together with advice to parents for a wide diapering, the importance of exercises during dressing of a child, and of course strictly phasing out the use of early child support (walker and stroller). Every orthopedic surgeon and every doctor meets this challenging efforts of bad inherited practices and efforts for an early child support. Pointing out this error is never enough.

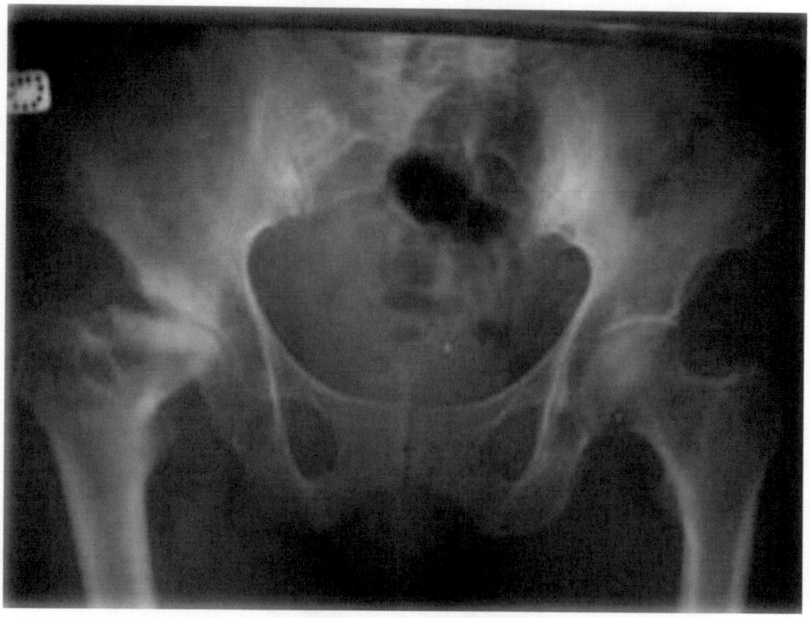

Figure 4. X-ray of the right neglected dysplastic hip and left healthy hip.

Abduction exercises for the hips suggest exercising approximately twenty times a day, each time you change a baby. These measures should be applied to every child as a mean of prevention.

Orthopedic briefs have almost been abandoned in practice, at our clinic as well. Its disadvantage lies in the fact that they can exacerbate harmful effect in the case of increased tension of adductor muscles.

Pavlik harness is a great way to treat DDH in the early months. Pavlik harnesses have the advantage of causing nonviolent reposition of the hip joint, and in addition, dynamically stimulate the development of joint elements. They can be used for the reduction, retention, and as an agent which enhances the maturation of the child hip. When we use them for reduction (reposition of the head in the acetabulum) the child is allowed to have small movements in the harness with basic abduction-flexion position. To encourage retention, we advise the use of tightly closed belts on the harness (pay attention to neurocirculatory status), while in the use for enhancing hip maturation we recommend the application as for a reduction but with no possibility of flexion in the hip. Reposition is achieved by abduction apparatus in flexion greater than 90 and abduction up to 50° (**Figures 5** and **6**).

Indications:

- primary DDH treatment at an early age; and
- continuation of treatment after the achievement repositioning with other method.

Application of the belt is made exclusively by a doctor in the presence of mother, but here we also must emphasize the importance of quality training of nurses to monitor the whole process.

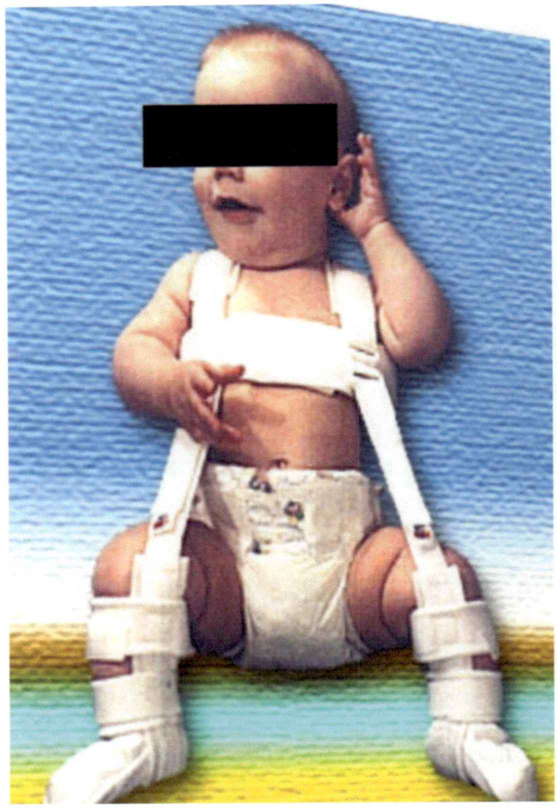

Figure 5. A child with Pavlik harness.

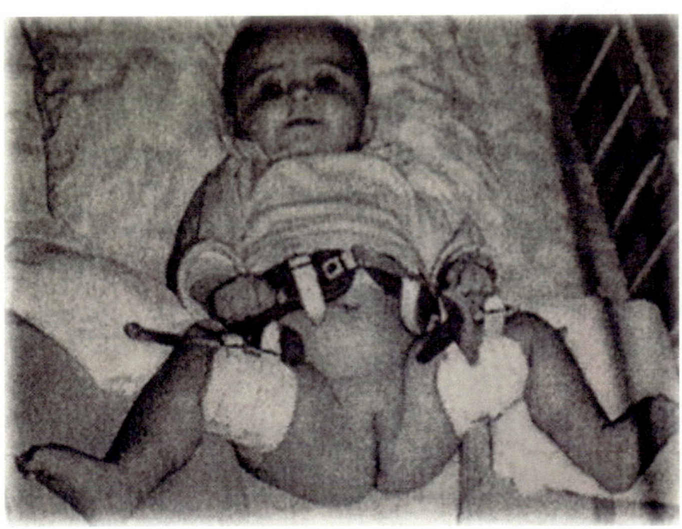

Figure 6. Apart from Pavlik harness, Hilger-Reiner apparatus is widely used in practice as well.

http://dx.doi.org/10.5772/67481

2.4.1. *Traction techniques*

Continuous traction aims to gradually progressively stretch the shortened soft tissues and to center the hip head in acetabulum, with the gradual adaptation of vascular and neurological elements.

Continuous traction is always carried out at the hospital. Here we should mention the position in which the reposition always takes place, and that is abduction and internal rotation.

There are two types of traction:

- overhead traction; and
- longitudinal traction according to Morel.

Overhead traction was first presented in the year 1955 in USA by Craig et al., and in Germany in the year 1956 by H. Mau and Dorr. Hips are flexed at the angle of 110° or more, while the abduction position is negligible (**Figure 7**). Abduction is increased very gently over the next 4 weeks, although the expansion is not recommended in the first 7 days. What occurs during this period is adaptation of adductor muscles and neurovascular net. Starting weight should not exceed 0.5–1 kg, depending on the age of the child. Mittelmeier reported 90% success with this method of repositioning. Essentially, we do not suggest a load increase over one-fifth of the body weight. Increasing the load to one-fourth of the body weight in order to enforce reposition has failed results [5].

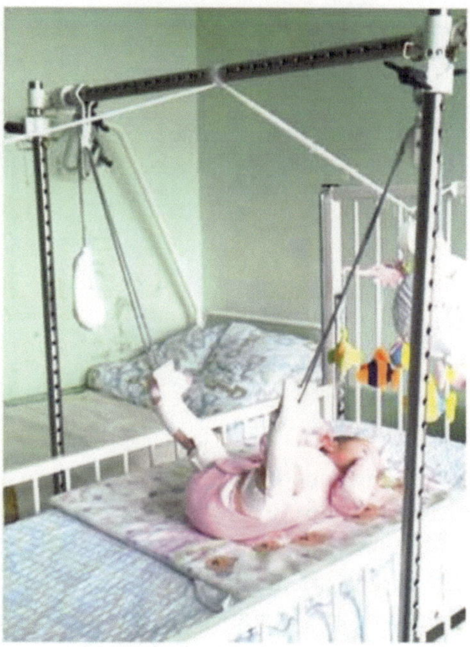

Figure 7. Risser traction is not only used before the apparatus application, but also as a part of preoperative patient preparation.

Longitudinal traction was displayed by Pravaz in 1874, and H. Mau and Dorr in Germany also presented this method and set rule that each closed reduction of luxated hip without preliminary traction represents the malpractice of the physician.

Elastic adhesive bandages are used to achieve the reduction. We recommend it to children of 12 months and to apply it in light flexion. Only after X-rays, if it shows the femoral head lowered below the level of the roof of acetabulum, we can begin easy abduction. If a physician is satisfied with reposition and stability of the hip, we suggest placing a child in vertical position and applying abduction apparatus for the walking below 60°. If the reduction is not stable, we recommend immobilizing the child with cast bandage in a reduced position.

We emphasize that the cast immobilization is done in the human position, which is the position of the upper leg abduction of 45°, 100 degrees of flexion with neutral rotation (**Figure 8**).

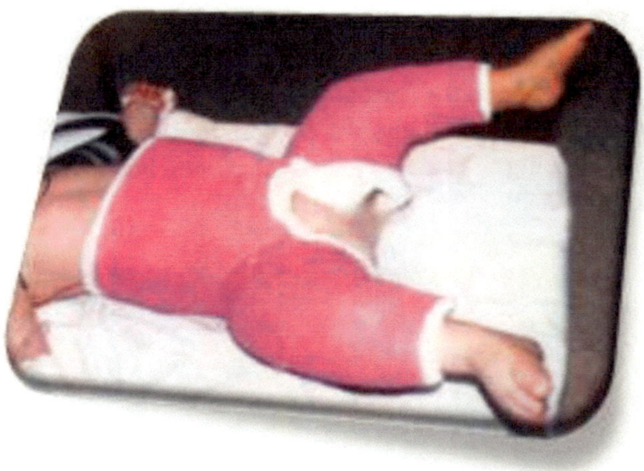

Figure 8. Cast shorts.

3. Conclusion

Hip ultrasonography as a screening method represents the most efficient and the cheapest method in detection of DDH where, with conservative treatment, great results can be achieved with no need for additional surgical intervention [6, 7]. This type of treatment represents relief for a patient, its' parents, medical personnel, and the society, in general. Because of this fact, appropriate and on-time cooperation among gynecologists, neonatologists, pediatricians, radiologists, and orthopedic surgeons is extremely important for early detection of DDH and the beginning of the conservative treatment [8].

http://dx.doi.org/10.5772/67481

Author details

Ismet Gavrankapetanović* and Adnan Papović

*Address all correspondence to: ismetcap@ortotrauma.com.ba

Clinic for Orthopedics and Traumatology, University Clinical Center Sarajevo, Sarajevo, Bosnia and Herzegovina

References

[1] Graf R. Is DDH still a problem. Arch Bone Jt Surg. 2014;March(2(1):2–3).

[2] Graf R, Mohajer M, Plattner F. Hip sonography update. Quality – management, catastrophes – tips and tricks. Med Ultrason. 2013;Dec(15(4):299–303).

[3] Graf R. The use of ultrasonography in developmental dysplasia of the hip. Acta Orthop Traumatol Turc. 2007;(41(Suppl 1):6–13).

[4] Stiegler H, Hafner E, Schuchter K, Engel A, Graf R. A sonographic study of perinatal hip development: from 34 weeks of gestation to 6 weeks of age. J Pediatr Orthop B. 2003;Nov(12(6):365–368).

[5] Burian M, Dungl P, Chomiak J, Oštadal M, Frydrychova M. Efficiency of conservative treatment by overhead traction in developmental dysplasia of the hip. Acta Chir Orthop Traumatol Cech. 2010;Oct(77(5):371–377).

[6] Dias JJ, Thomas IH, Lamont AC, Mody BS, Thompson JR. The reliability of ultrasonographic assessment of neonatal hips. J Bone Joint Surg. 1993;(75(3):479–482).

[7] Leonhardi A, Reither M. Ultrasound screening of newborn infants. Uses and role in routine diagnosis. Klinische Pediatrie. 1993;(205(6):383–388).

[8] Matasović T, Strinković B. Dječija ortopedija. Zagreb: Školska knjiga; 1986.

Chapter 4

Pelvic Osteotomies for Developmental Dysplasia of the Hip

Chunho Chen, Ting-Ming Wang and Ken N. Kuo

Additional information is available at the end of the chapter

http://dx.doi.org/10.5772/67516

Abstract

Treatment of developmental dysplasia of the hip (DDH) is based on concentric reducibility of the femoral head, patient age and the status of triradiate cartilage. Patients in walking age are indicated for pelvic osteotomy to correct the dysplastic acetabulum. Salter innominate osteotomy and Pemberton osteotomy are the most widely used procedures to treat the developmental dysplasia of the hip in early childhood. Although short-term results of the pelvic osteotomies are reported well, some long-term sequalae such as coxa valga caused by Kalamchi type II osteonecrosis of the femoral head, leg length discrepancy and impingement of hip may occur.

Keywords: developmental dysplasia of the hip (DDH), Pemberton, salter, pelvic osteotomy, open reduction

1. Introduction

Developmental dysplasia of the hip (DDH) is one of the most important issues in paediatric orthopaedics which include dysplastic, subluxated or dislocated hips. The principle of the treatment is to achieve a congruent and concentrically reduced hip, eventually to prevent premature osteoarthritis of hip. Many treatment options have been developed to achieve the goal, which varied from close reduction to several kinds of combined osteotomies. The choice of treatment for DDH is age-related with consideration of specific pathologic conditions. Although the minimum age at which an acetabular osteotomy should be done is still a controversy, it is generally accepted that DDH in a child of walking age should be treated with acetabuloplasty. This chapter focuses on the Salter innominate osteotomy and Pemberton osteotomy.

2. Pelvic osteotomies

There are numerous types of pelvic osteotomies to treat the dysplastic hips. To determine which osteotomy is the most appropriate, we should consider concentric reducibility of the femoral head, patient age and the status of triradiate cartilage (**Figure 1**).

For the patients with late diagnosed DDH, the reconstructive osteotomy for dysplastic acetabulum is indicated only when the femoral head can be concentrically reduced. Salter innominate osteotomy and Pemberton osteotomy are the most commonly used procedures for children younger than 7 years old [1].

Salter osteotomy and Pemberton acetabuloplasty are common procedures for deficient acetabulum in developmental dysplasia of the hip (DDH). Salter osteotomy redirects the entire acetabulum following a complete trans-iliac osteotomy, while Pemberton acetabuloplasty modifies the shape of the acetabulum by hinging the horizontal branch of the triradiate cartilage following an incomplete osteotomy. The objectives of these two procedures are to improve the coverage of the femoral head for acetabular dysplasia.

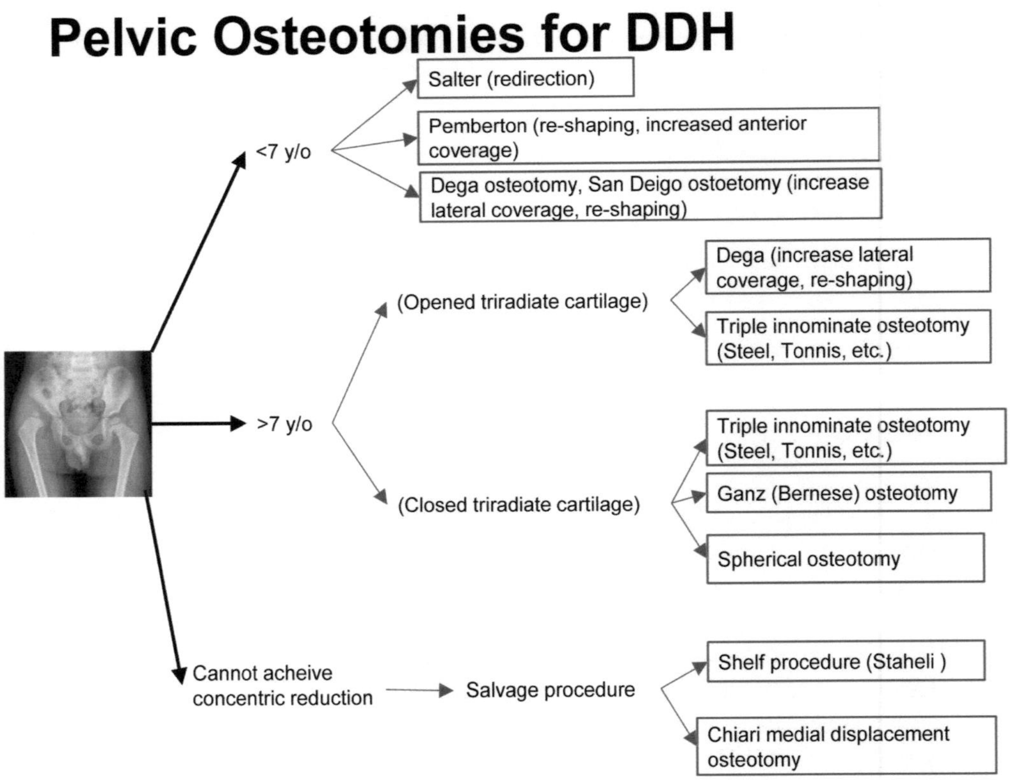

Figure 1. Varies types of pelvic osteotomies for DDH are indicated depending on the reduction concentricity, patient age and the status of triradiate cartilage.

http://dx.doi.org/10.5772/67516

The pericapsular acetabuloplasty, described by Pemberton in 1965, is a unique type of pelvic osteotomy. Through an incomplete cut in the ilium, this procedure can redirect the acetabulum to achieve correction of acetabular dysplasia. Pemberton's original study demonstrated a high rate of satisfactory results in children younger than 7 years of age. Later some authors have obtained a good result in older children when they applied one stage Pemberton acetabuloplasty and femoral shortening as a one-stage operation [2, 3]. In addition, to obtain correction of the acetabular dysplasia that is potentially greater than that achieved with the Salter osteotomy, the Pemberton osteotomy can be performed without the use of internal fixation. The objective of the surgery is to improve the anterolateral coverage of the femoral head. Adequate containment and a stable hip allow weight bearing and osseous remodelling of the dysplastic acetabulum.

In 1961, Salter described the innominate osteotomy for stabilizing the reduced hip by redirection of the acetabulum as a unit. The procedure was accomplished by a transverse osteotomy of the ilium perpendicular to the iliac axis from just above the anterior inferior iliac spine to the sciatic notch. It was designed to preserve the acetabular shape while correcting the abnormal anterolateral facing of the acetabulum in DDH. The pubic symphysis served as a rotating hinge and the acetabulum can be redirected to cover the anterolateral deficiency in a concentrically reduced hip after the osteotomy [4]. Salter and Dubos reported 93.6% excellent or good results in patients operated from 18 months to 4 years of age with no failures in a review of 15-year follow-up on 140 patients. In the 4–10-year-old age group, the results were excellent or good in only 56.7% [5]. Thus, the Salter osteotomy is not recommended in older children. This procedure is probably the most widely used pelvic osteotomy in the treatment of DDH. In comparison with the Pemberton osteotomy, the Salter's procedure seems relatively simple. However, its proper technical execution is not easy. The most common error that leads to a catastrophic outcome is failure to achieve a concentric reduction of the hip joint before innominate osteotomy.

3. Pre-OP evaluation

Complete clinical examination is necessary before surgery including inspection of walking pattern, skin folds of thigh and gluteal creases, and physical examination of both hips including range of motion (ROM) and reducibility of the hip. The affected lower limb is shorter than the healthy side. Children may walk on their toe to compensate the discrepancy of limb length. Some children may have Trendelenburg gait. Because the thigh length is shorter in the affected side due to dislocated hip, there will be more thigh skin folds than the healthy side (**Figure 2**). However, the extra thigh folds are common normal variants, especially for the young babies, and it is not the sufficient and necessary condition of the hip dislocation. Physical examination may reveal positive Allis' sign, which is appreciated by placing both hips flexion in 90° with full flexion of the knees and comparing the height of the knees (**Figure 3**). Positive Allis' sign indicate shortening of the affected limb but does not differentiate femur or tibia as the primary cause. Galeazzi's sign is comparing the height of the knees when both hips and knees are placed in 90–90° flexion, which is specifically indicating shortening of the femur.

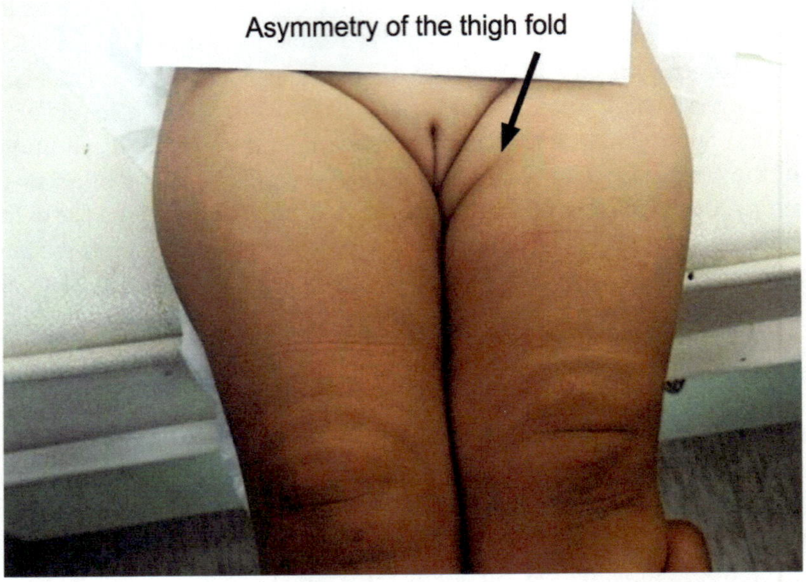

Figure 2. Asymmetry of thigh folds: With left hip dislocated, the skin fold of thigh is asymmetric due to apparent shortening of the lower limb on the left side.

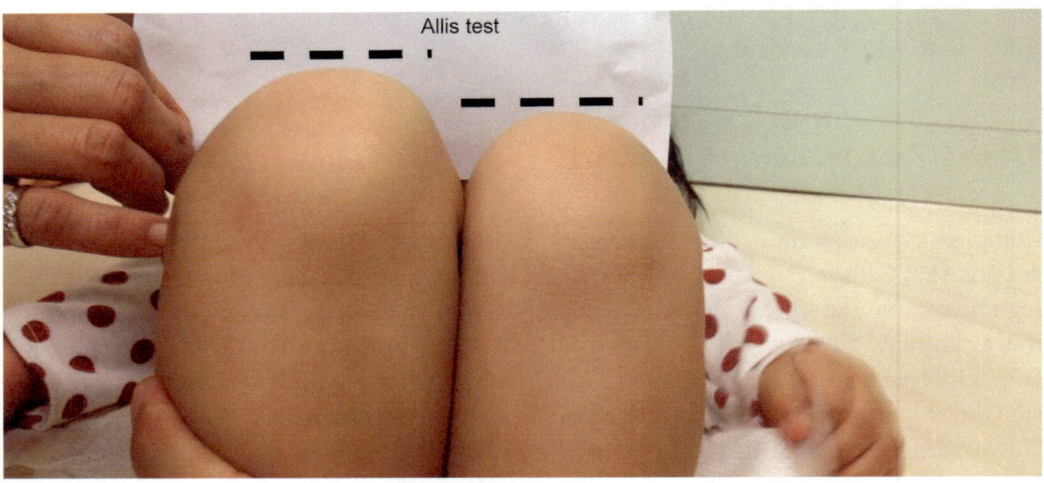

Figure 3. The affected limb is shorter than the normal side as demonstrated by different knee level when the child is lying supine on the examination table with the hips flexed 90° and knees fully flexed.

http://dx.doi.org/10.5772/67516

Complete radiographic examinations include a standing pelvis AP view, frog leg lateral view and false-profile radiographs to determine the severity of acetabular dysplasia and deformity of proximal femur.

Ortolani's and Barlow's test have high sensitivity and specificity under an experienced surgeon's hand. Sometimes those tests cannot be performed very well to an awake child. Usually, the tests will demonstrate clearly under general anaesthesia. Close reduction of the hip joint will be tried first after anaesthesia. The tension of hip adductor tendons should be evaluated after closed reduction of the hip joint. If adductor contracture is presented, adductor tenotomy can be done simultaneously.

Generally speaking, the children younger than 3 years old with simple dislocated hip can be treated by open reduction of hip joint and Pemberton osteotomy or Salter osteotomy alone. For those older than 3 years old, combined femoral osteotomy is often required to achieve stable reduction of the hip joint.

4. Surgical technique (open reduction of hip joint and Pemberton osteotomy)

4.1. Step 1: incision and surgical approach

- Pass the stockinette to wrap around the body and put the stockinette to the level of nipple first. It may facilitate the spica casting technique and avoid excessive manipulation of hip after surgery to prevent bone graft dislodgement or re-dislocation (**Figure 4**).
- Patient is placed in supine position and a small towel roll is placed under the ipsilateral buttock.
- Make a bikini incision just slightly medial to the iliac crest.
- Dissect the subcutaneous tissue and identify the muscle interval between the Sartorius and tensor fascia femoris muscles (**Figure 5**). The lateral femoral cutaneous nerve should be identified and protected which passes distally and laterally beneath the deep fascia in this inter-muscular interval. Retract lateral femoral cutaneous nerve medially after it is well mobilized proximally and distally.
- Expose the iliac crest. Releasing the external oblique muscle fibres on the iliac crest facilitates exposure of the cartilaginous iliac apophysis. Identify the anterior superior iliac spine.
- Hold the iliac crest by thumb and index finger to define the margin of the iliac crest and sharply incise the iliac apophysis exactly in the midline (**Figure 6**). Strip off the iliac apophysis with a periosteal elevator to expose the ilium sub-periosteally both medially and laterally. Pack gauze sponges on both inner and outer table of the ilium to facilitate sub-periosteal dissection and provide haemostasis.

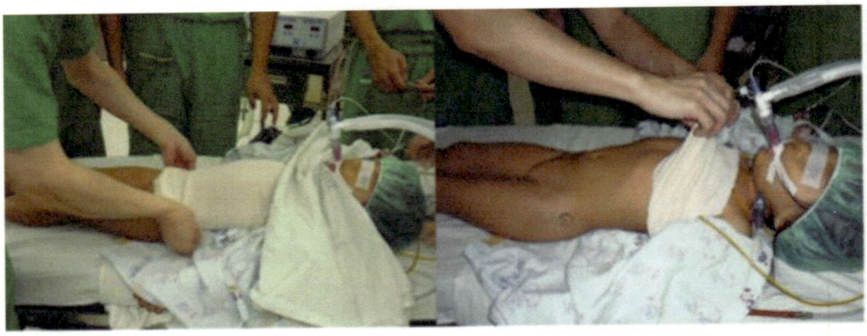

Figure 4. The stockinette is prepared and placed at the level of nipple line to facilitate the postoperative spica casting procedure.

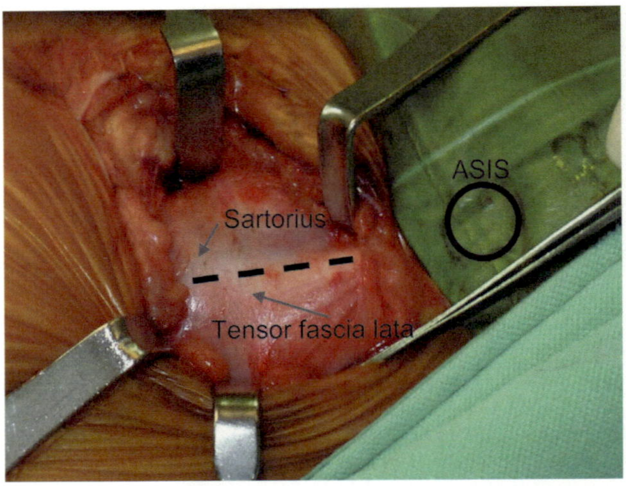

Figure 5. Identify the muscle interval between sartorius and tensor fascia lata muscles. ASIS = anterior superior iliac spine.

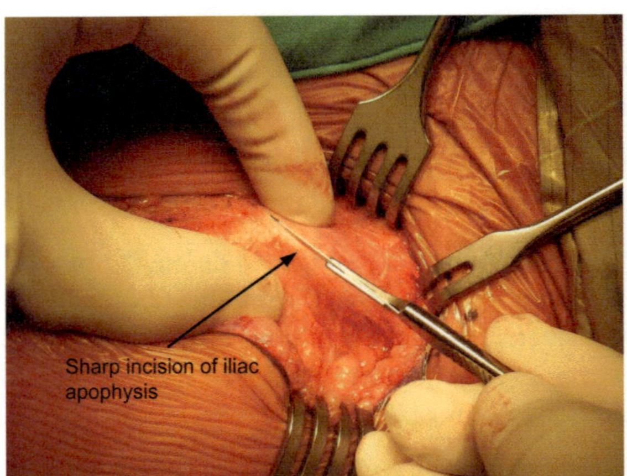

Figure 6. The iliac crest cartilaginous apophysis is split sharply, with the thumb and the index finger as the guide for thickness and direction of the iliac wing.

http://dx.doi.org/10.5772/67516

- The anterior inferior iliac spine (AIIS) is exposed by sub-periosteal elevation of the hip abductors from the outer cortex of the ilium.

4.2. Step 2: rectus femoris and iliopsoas identification and tenotomy

- The straight head of the rectus femoris muscle is exposed at its origin on the AIIS. The rectus femoris tendon is transected close to the anterior inferior iliac spine. A short stump is left for later tendon reattachment. Protect and preserve the ascending branch of the anterior femoral circumflex artery in the surgical field to protect the blood supply of the femoral head.
- The psoas tendon is located beneath the iliacus muscle and can be identified by blunt dissection of the iliacus muscle belly medial to the ilium at the level of the anterior pelvic rim. Tendinous part of the Iliopsoas muscle is released (**Figure 7**). Care must be taken to protect the femoral neurovascular bundle, which is located immediately medial and slightly anterior to the iliacus muscle. A blunt retractor is useful in protecting the femoral neurovascular bundle in the surgical field.
- The edge of the acetabulum and the reflected head of the rectus femoris muscle are clearly identified. Find the margin of the joint capsule at the acetabular rim and expose the anterior aspect of entire joint capsule. The capsule may be redundant and adherent to the ilium as a result of femoral head dislocation. Use a periosteal elevator to strip off any soft tissue from the anterior aspect of the ilium to reveal the junction of the hip capsule and cartilaginous labrum.

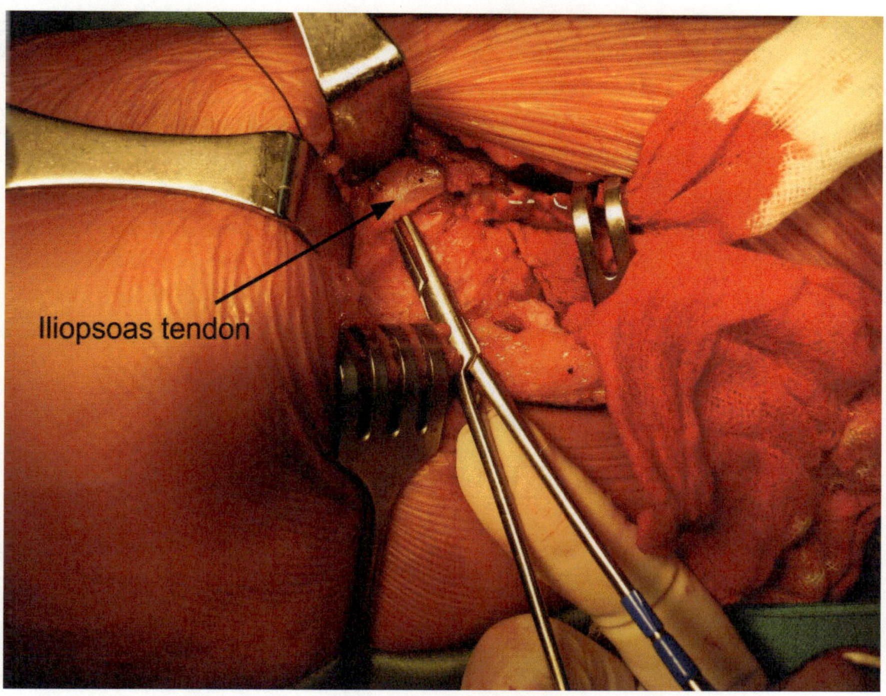

Figure 7. The iliopsoas tendon is identified at the pelvic rim, and the tendinous portion is divided, leaving the muscular portion intact.

4.3. Step 3: open reduction of dislocated hip joint and ilium osteotomy

Perform an open reduction, check hip stability, make medial and lateral cut lines and complete the osteotomy.

- For a dislocated hip, open reduction is needed. A T-shaped capsulotomy near the acetabular rim, including the upper and lower margins of the hip capsule, is done (**Figure 8**). The stem of the T-shaped capsulotomy is parallel to the femoral neck and is slightly superior to avoid a small inferior capsular flap, which may make the capsulorrhaphy difficult. The ligamentum teres are cut sharply, and all of the fibro-fatty tissues (pulvinar tissue) are removed from the true acetabulum (**Figure 9**). The transverse acetabular ligament is seated in the inferior part of the true acetabulum. The tension of the ligament is palpated by the finger and released by scissors. The tension of the ligament is tested again by palpation to confirm complete release of the transverse acetabular ligament. The remaining transverse acetabular ligament can impede complete reduction of the femoral head.

- The femoral head is gently reduced into the acetabulum under direct vision. The stability of the hip joint is checked in a neutral position as well as in abduction and internal rotation. If the hip is unstable in a neutral position but is stable in abduction and internal rotation, a Pemberton acetabuloplasty is indicated. If hip stability cannot be maintained even in abduction and internal rotation, an additional proximal femoral varus and/or rotational osteotomy should be considered.

- The gauze sponges are removed on either side of the iliac bone. All of the bleeders from the iliac wing or from the periosteum are checked. Pemberton osteotomy can begin once haemostasis is achieved. The sciatic notch is identified first with a small periosteal elevator and the adjacent soft tissue, including the sciatic nerve are protected with two small Hohmann retractors. The medial iliac cut line is outlined with the electrocautery tip. Using a small straight osteotome, begin the medial cut line about 1–1.5 cm above the superior hip joint line and curve it inferiorly and posteriorly, aiming at the sciatic notch. The cut line extends halfway to the sciatic notch and ends at the ridge of the pelvic inlet of the ilium. The lateral cut line has the same starting point as the medial cut. With the medial cut line as a reference, use the same osteotome to make the lateral cut line along the joint capsule. (**Figure 10**).

- A wider, curved osteotome is used to complete the osteotomy. The medial and lateral cut lines are connected with a curved osteotome (**Figure 11**). As this osteotomy advances, the osteotome is pushed against the distal fragment to check the degree of downward displacement. If the osteotomy site opens more than 2–3 cm that means that the distal fragment is hinging on the triradiate cartilage and there is no further advancement of the osteotome needed. If the opening is insufficient, osteotome should be advanced slightly and the amount of osteotomy opening is checked again until the opening is adequate.

http://dx.doi.org/10.5772/67516

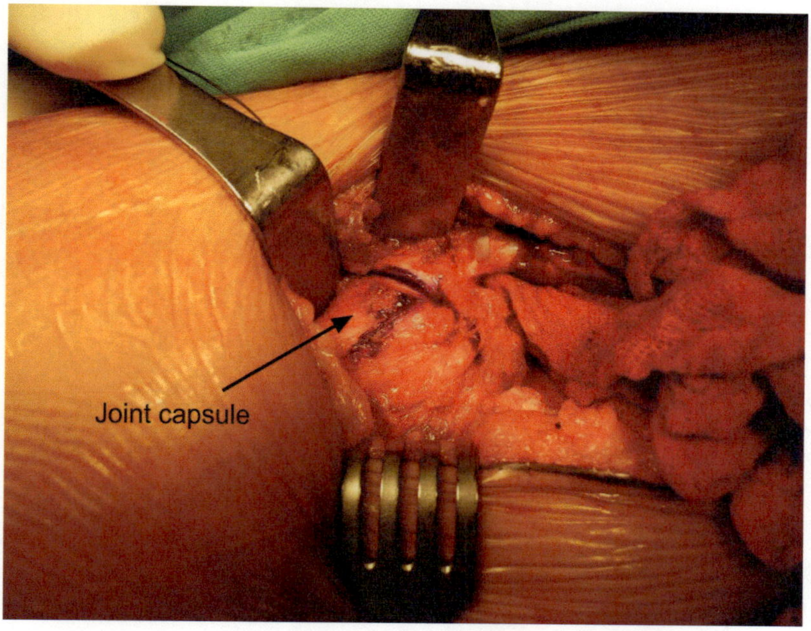

Figure 8. Capsular incision outline with the stem of the T parallel with the femoral neck.

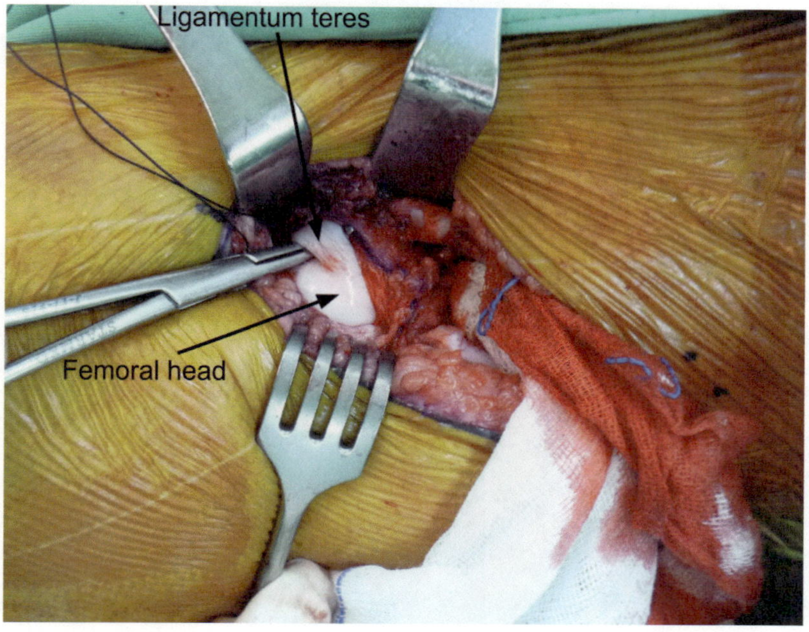

Figure 9. After T-capsulotomy, dislocated femoral head and redundant ligamentum teres are visualized.

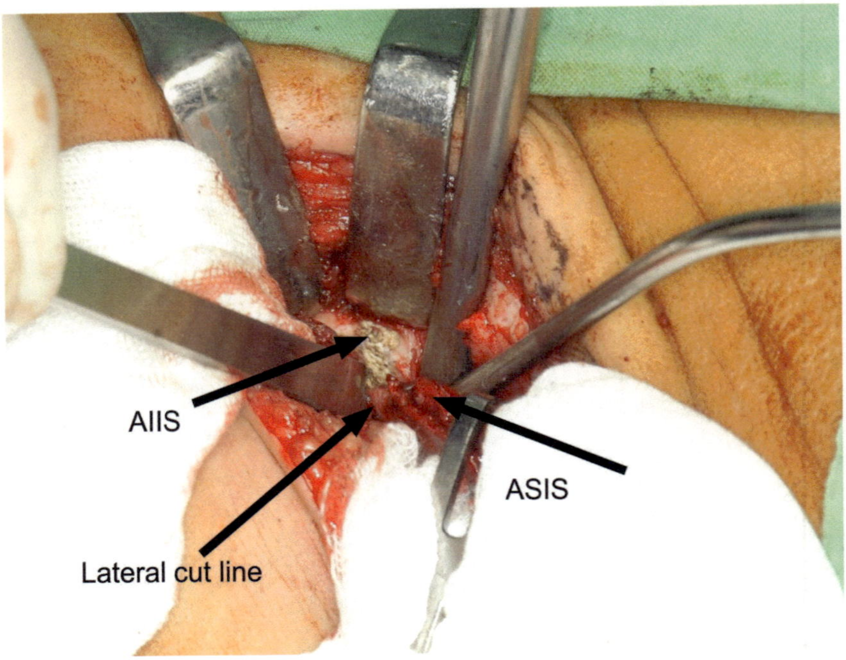

Figure 10. Lateral cut line starts between the ASIS and AIIS.

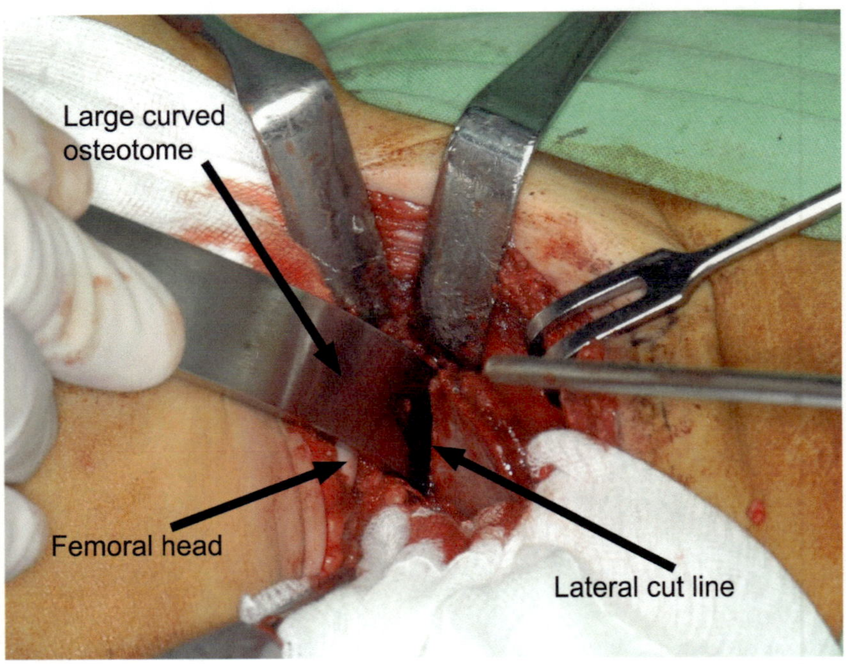

Figure 11. Complete the osteotomy with a large-curved osteotome.

http://dx.doi.org/10.5772/67516

4.4. Step 4: insert the bone graft

Harvest the graft, position the reduced hip joint, insert the bone graft, repair the capsule and close the wound.

- A triangular-shaped iliac crest bone graft is harvested from the iliac wing with a bone cutter or an oscillating saw.
- With the femoral head in reduced position, a towel roll is placed underneath the knee to help maintain the hip in an abducted and flexed position.
- Two towel clips are used to hold the superior and inferior osteotomy fragments, respectively. The inferior fragment is manipulated anteriorly and inferiorly to cover the femoral head. Then insert the triangularly shaped bone graft into the osteotomy opening site. Usually, when the triangular iliac bone graft is stably seated in the osteotomy site, no internal fixation is needed (**Figure 12**). If the bone graft is not stable, fixation with one or two Kirschner wires may be necessary.
- The hip capsule is repaired by bringing the two flaps of the T-capsulotomy to the acetabular flap of the capsule. The tendon of the straight head of the rectus femoris muscle is reattached to the anterior inferior iliac spine. Suture the iliac apophysis over the ilium and close the wound.

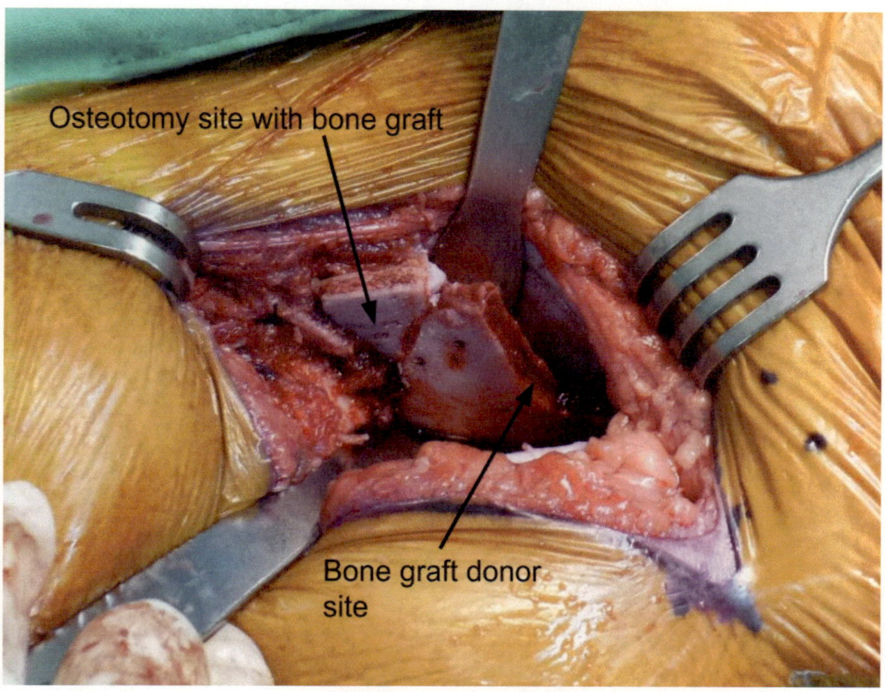

Figure 12. Bone graft is inserted after opening the osteotomy site.

4.5. Step 5: post-operative management

A hip spica cast is applied after the wound closure. Both hips are held in about 20° of flexion, 30° of abduction each, and neutral or slight internal rotation to stabilize the hip while the cast is applied. For patients undergoing a simple Pemberton osteotomy, the spica cast is worn for four weeks. For patients with combined open reduction of the hip, the spica cast is applied for 6 weeks, followed by use, for 4 weeks, of a hip abduction brace or an 'A cast' (a bilateral cylinder cast with a spreader bar, holding each hip at 30° abduction) [6, 7].

5. Surgical technique (Salter innominate Osteotomy)

5.1. Step 1: surgical approach and hip joint exploration

The same skin incision and surgical approach as previously described in this chapter for Pemberton osteotomy are used to explore the dislocated hip joint.

5.2. Step 2: innominate osteotomy

Expose the inner and outer table of the ilium sub-periosteally until sciatic notch is totally visualized. Pass an Ethibond suture with a right angled clamp through the sciatic notch and grasp the Ethibon suture with a Kelly clamp. Tie the Gigli saw with the Ethibon suture as a guide to pass through the sciatic notch (**Figure 13**). Place two Hohmann retractors or Rang retractors

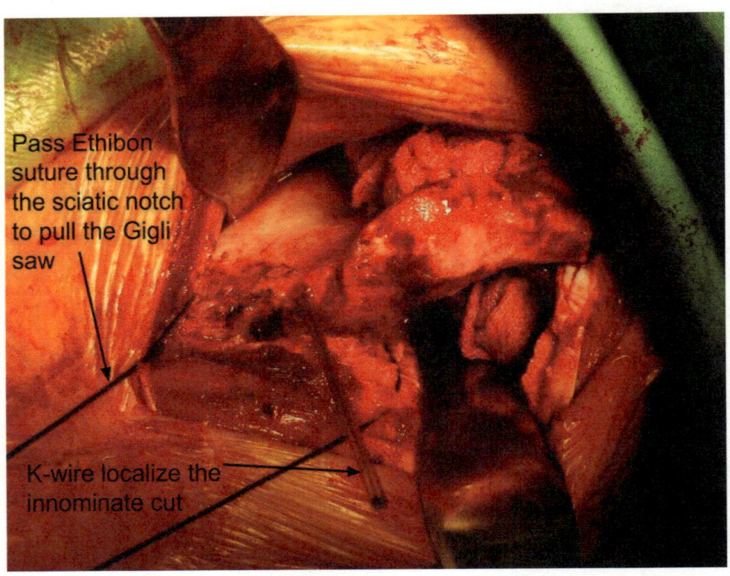

Figure 13. Both tables of the ilium are exposed sub-periosteally and place the blunt Hohmann retractor at the sciatic notch to protect the soft tissue during procedure. Passing a No. 5. Ethibon suture through sciatic notch to pull the Gigli saw can facilitate the procedure, also protect the adjacent soft tissues while passing Gigli saw.

during passage of the Gigli saw to protect the sciatic nerve. The complete osteotomy is done with Gigli saw, starting from sciatic notch and emerging in between anterior superior iliac spine and anterior inferior iliac spine.

5.3. Step 3: insert the iliac bone graft and fix with K-wires

Harvest a wedge-shaped iliac crest bone graft from the iliac wing with a bone cutter or a power saw. With the hip in frog leg position, hold the two fragments of ilium with towel clips and open the osteotomy site with distal fragment pulling towards inferior and lateral position. The distal fragment should be held as far posterior as possible to prevent fracture of the distal fragment during opening of the osteotomy site. Then insert the triangularly shaped bone graft into the osteotomy opening site. Fix the fragments and the bone graft with two or more K-wires. Confirm the pins position with intraoperative radiograph and make sure not to penetrate the hip joint. Check the stability of the hip joint and the stability of fixation with passively moving the hip joint. Carefully palpate any crepitus or clicking which may indicate the penetration of the K-wire into the hip joint.

5.4. Post-operative management

Apply the hip spica cast as previously described in this chapter for Pemberton osteotomy. The hip spica cast should be continued for 6 weeks. After removal of the spica cast, abduction brace is applied for 4 weeks. Weight bearing or walking under abduction brace is allowed (**Figures 14–16**).

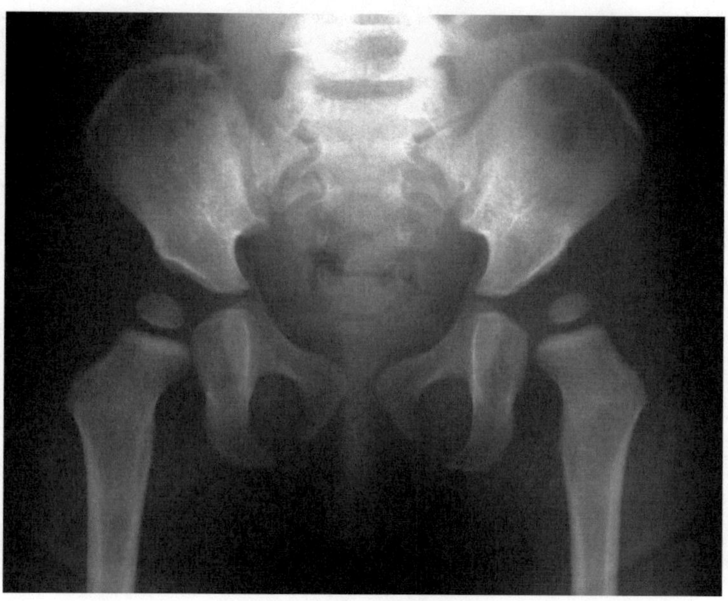

Figure 14. A 16-month-old girl with left-hip dysplasia and lateral subluxation. Note the Shenton's line is disrupted and the acetabular index is 50° in the left side.

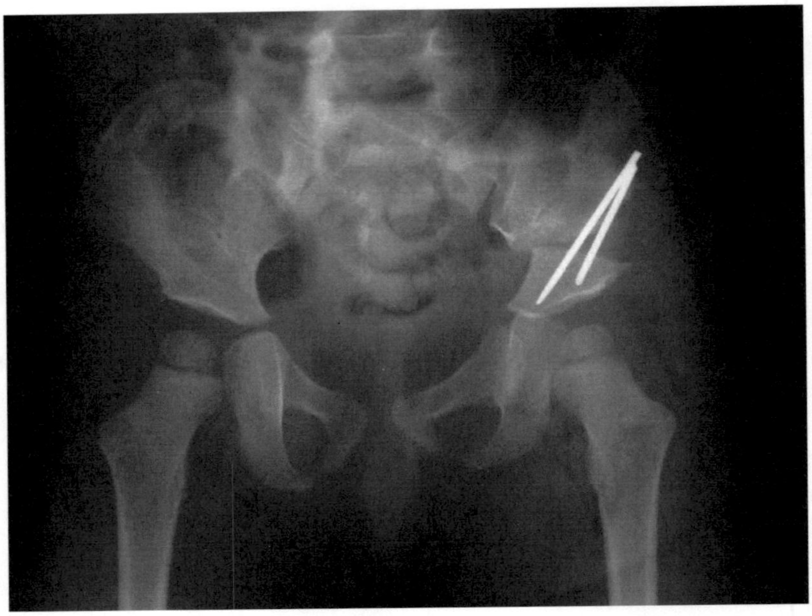

Figure 15. Radiograph after Salter Osteotomy and internal fixation with two K-wires when the patient was 22 months old. The Shenton's line is smooth in each side.

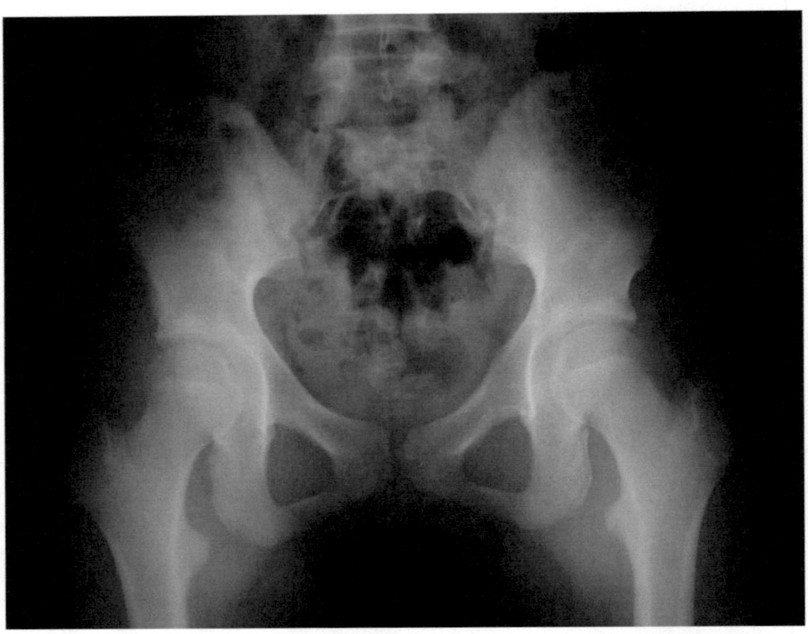

Figure 16. Final radiograph, taken when the patient was 13 years old, reveals well-developed hips. The patient was totally symptom free.

http://dx.doi.org/10.5772/67516

5.5. Complications

The surgeon should pay attention to every detail of the procedure to avoid the complications. Sciatic nerve injury is a devastating complication during osteotomy. The iliac wing bone cut should always be protected by the instruments such as Hohmann retractors or Rang retractors during the passage of the Gigli saw in the sciatic notch. Loss of fixation sometimes occurs if the K-wires are not placed in the appropriate position. K-wire penetration into the hip joint or even into the femoral head should be prevented by intraoperative radiographs.

6. Surgical technique (combined procedure for high dislocation in patients with developmental dysplasia of the hip)

A late presentation of DDH in patients older than 3 years old often is characterized by high dislocation and irreducible joint. It is more common that children with bilateral dislocation are brought to orthopaedic surgeon's attention at older age. They are usually in higher Tönnis grade than patients with unilateral dysplasia [8]. A combined procedure including open reduction, femoral-shortening osteotomy and an acetabular procedure is often necessary to obtain a desirable result in children of walking age who have a high-riding hip dislocation. The combined procedure with femoral shortening, although technically demanding, helps prevent excessive force that hinders concentric reduction and decreases the risk of complications related to open reduction, especially re-dislocation and osteonecrosis, which are common in older children. In case with severe dysplasia, acetabulum may be globally deficient. For the patient with globally deficient acetabulum, a careful planning of combined femoral shortening, derotation osteotomy or flexion-extension osteotomy is required to prevent posterior dislocation of the hip after surgery [9].

6.1. Step 1: surgical approach and hip joint exploration

The same skin incision and surgical approach as previously described in this chapter for Pemberton osteotomy was used to explore the dislocated hip joint.

6.2. Step 2: femoral head reducibility

Reduce the femoral head with traction and check the soft-tissue tension. If the femoral head is reducible, place it into the acetabulum under direct vision and test the hip stability in a neutral position as well as in abduction and internal rotation by pushing the femoral head in a cephalad direction. If the hip is unstable in a neutral position but is stable in abduction and internal rotation, a Pemberton acetabuloplasty is indicated. When the femoral head is not reducible or is under great tension when reduced, a femoral shortening osteotomy should be performed.

6.3. Step 3: femoral osteotomy

Start the second incision from the lower tip of the greater trochanter and extend distally. The length of the incision, usually about 5–6 cm, depends on the length of the implant used for fixation of the osteotomy site and the required amount of shortening of the femur. Expose the femoral shaft by splitting the tensor fasciae latae and elevate the vastus lateralis off the lateral inter-muscular septum, coagulating perforating branches of profundus femoris vessel as needed. Expose the greater trochanter base; make an L-shaped incision at the proximal origin of the vastus lateralis muscle (**Figure 17**). Cut and elevate the periosteum longitudinally, and insert Chandler retractors under the sub-periosteal space to expose the femoral shaft. Insert a Steinmann pin into the femoral neck perpendicular to the femoral shaft just below the greater trochanteric apophysis under fluoroscopic guidance. This pin will serve as a joystick for checking the femoral head position. Insert a second Steinmann pin in the projected distal femoral segment in the same rotation plane and perpendicular to the shaft of the femur for rotational guidance. Make another longitudinal mark on the anterior aspect of the proximal part of the shaft as an additional orientation marker for femoral rotation (**Figure 18**). Make a transverse mark with an oscillating saw on the femoral shaft at the lower level of the lesser trochanter under fluoroscopic guidance as a marker of the osteotomy site (**Figure 19**). Using a four-hole DCP (dynamic compression plate) as a template, make two pre-drilled holes at the proximal end for better fixation alignment later. Divide the bone with an oscillating saw at the previously marked site. Make sure that the periosteum is well stripped so that you can manipulate the femoral head position with the proximal Steinmann pin as a joystick.

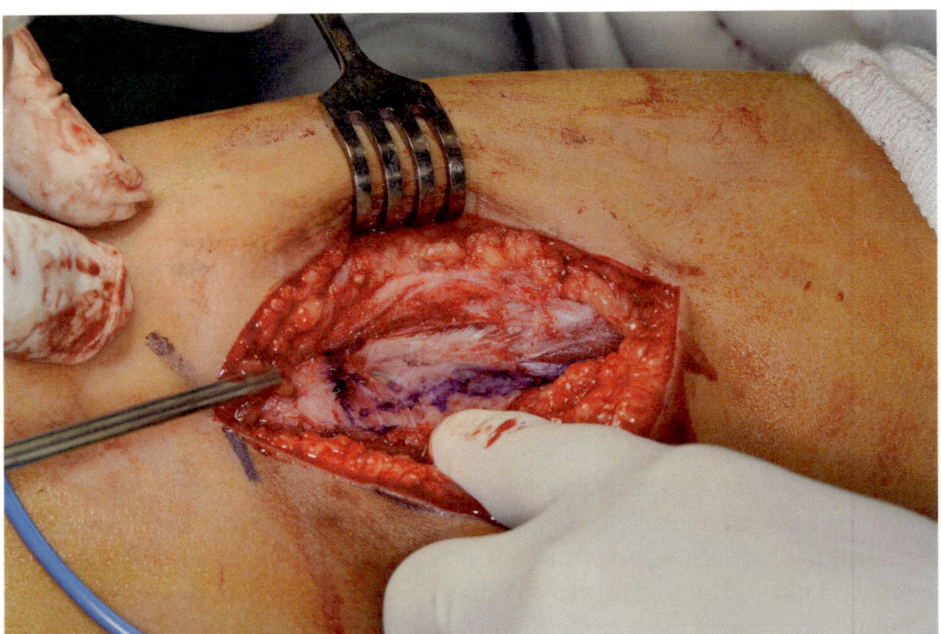

Figure 17. Marking for vastus lateralis incision.

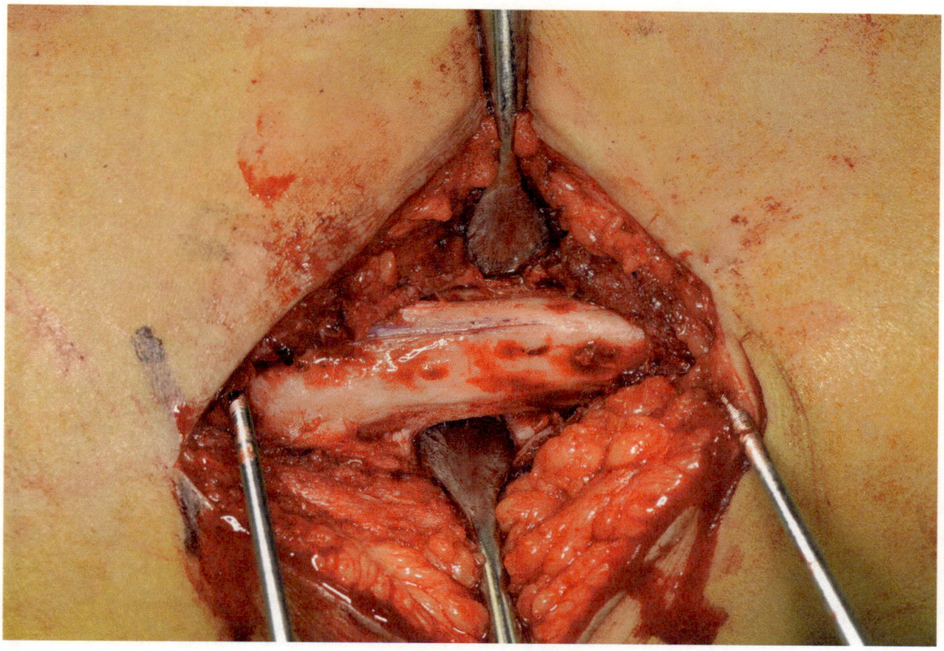

Figure 18. Insert parallel Steinman pins for rotational orientation. Marked the longitudinal rotation mark on the anterior aspect of femoral shaft.

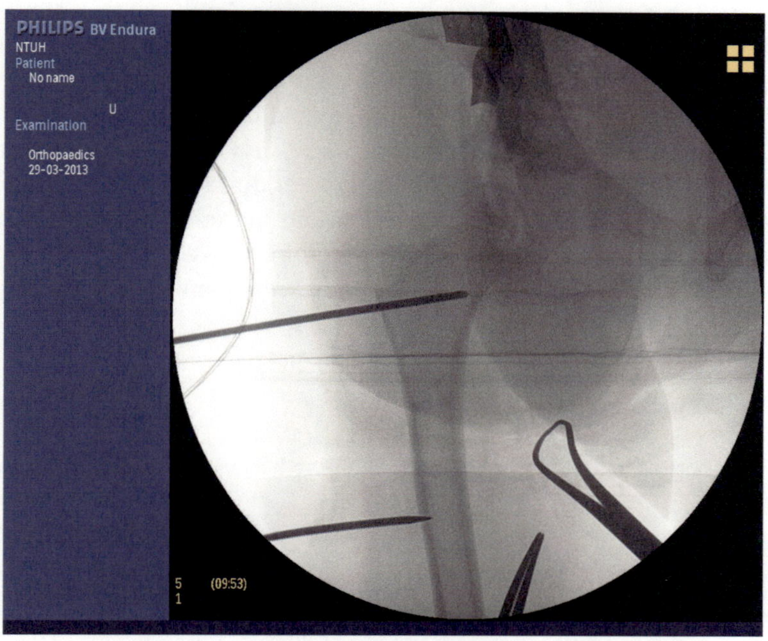

Figure 19. Fluoroscopic view showing two Steinman pins in parallel position. Marking of the osteotomy site under c-arm guided.

6.4. Step 4: hip joint stability

Manipulate the proximal Steinmann pin to reduce the femoral head under direct vision. Check the coverage of the femoral head and the stability of the reduction and assess the necessity for rotational osteotomy and pelvic osteotomy. If the femoral head cannot be reduced in a stable manner or the reduction cannot be maintained unless the proximal fragment is in internal rotation and/or abduction, an additional proximal femoral derotational osteotomy and/or varus osteotomy should be considered. Once the optimal position is achieved, have the assistance to hold the femoral head in an optimum position by holding the proximal Steinmann pin and return to the femoral shaft exposure.

6.5. Step 5: femoral shortening

Estimate the amount of shortening from the preoperative standing pelvic anteroposterior radiograph, and measure the amount of step-off at the broken Shenton line. The amount of shortening depends on the height of the dislocation; generally, 1–2 cm is required for neglected developmental dysplasia of the hip in a patient between 3 and 5 years old and 2–3 cm is required for patients between 5 and 8 years old. Holding the knee in neutral position with gentle tension, in correct rotational axis and angulation, measure the amount of overlapping. The length of overlapping of the bone ends is the amount of femoral shortening required (**Figures 20** and **21**). Resect the shortening section from the proximal end of the distal fragment of the femur (**Figure 22**). Reduce the femoral head into the acetabulum again, using the Steinmann pin as a joystick. Bring both ends of the femoral shaft together with the femoral head held in a reduced position by the assistant. Apply a pre-contoured four-hole DCP or locking plate on the reduced fragments with two holes on the proximal fragment and two holes on the distal fragment (**Figure 23**). Insert the proximal-fragment screws into the predrilled holes first. Use a reduction clamp to hold the distal segment and the plate in the desirable position. Insert the distal-fragment screws and complete the internal fixation in ideal position. Check the stability of the hip joint under direct vision, or with fluoroscopy if necessary, through the hip range of motion. At this time, the amount of rotation corrected can be seen from the relative rotation of two Steinmann pins viewed from caudally (**Figure 24**). Do not place the distal fragment in excessive external rotation if an acetabular procedure is contemplated.

6.6. Step 6: Pemberton acetabuloplasty

Perform the Pemberton osteotomy and insert the iliac bone graft as previously described in this chapter.

6.7. Post-operative management

Apply a one and a half hip spica cast with the hip in 30° of abduction, 20° of flexion and neutral to 10° of internal rotation. Remove the spica cast after 6 weeks. A hip abduction brace is then used full time for 6 weeks and at night for an additional 3 months.

http://dx.doi.org/10.5772/67516

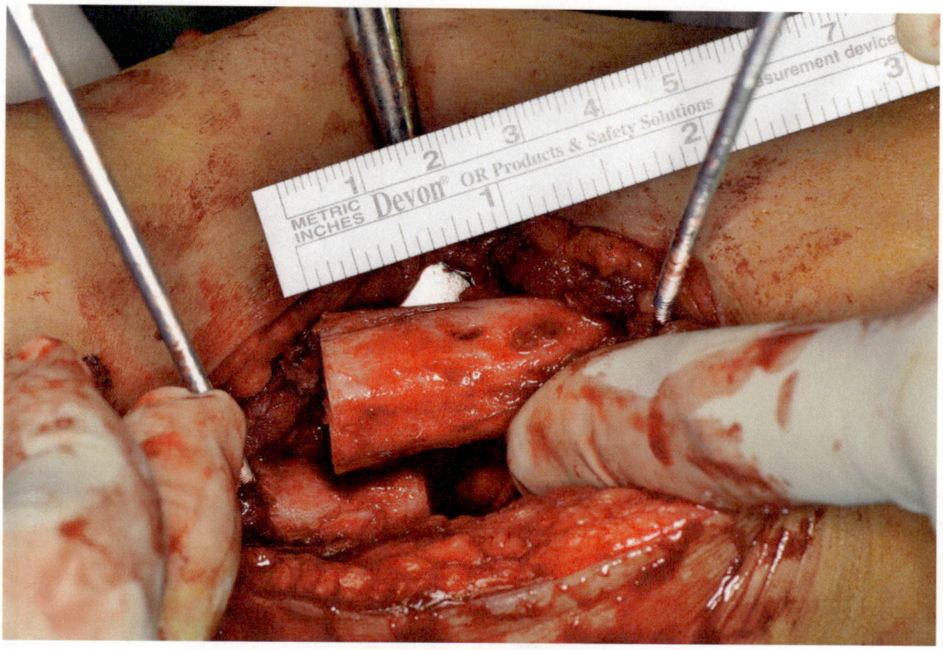

Figure 20. The amount of overlapping while the femoral head is in the reduced position is the amount of femoral shortening required.

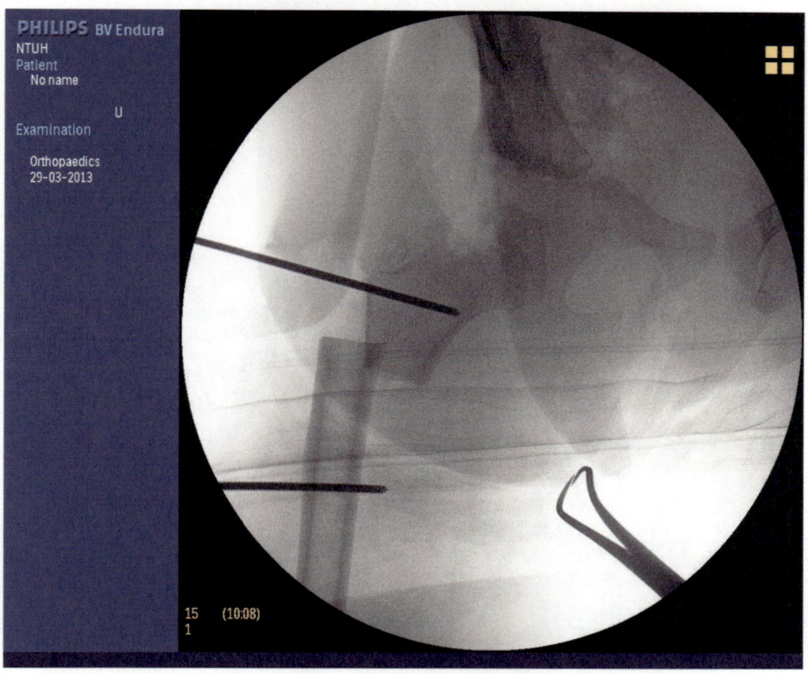

Figure 21. C-arm view shows the amount of shortening required while the femoral head is in a reduced position.

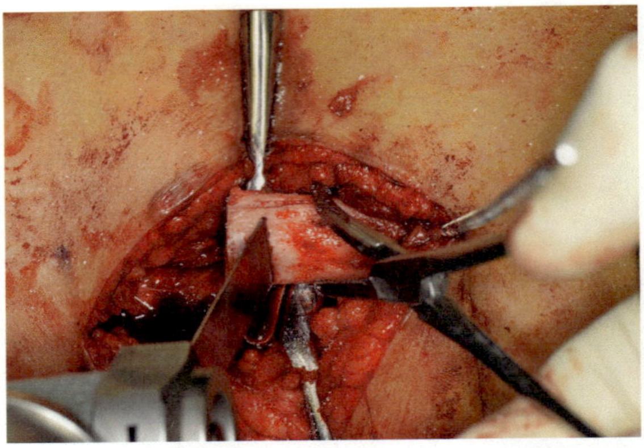

Figure 22. The fragment is removed from the proximal end of the distal fragment.

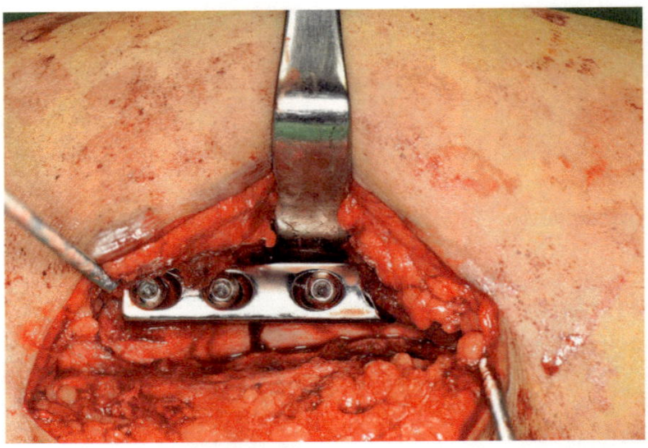

Figure 23. Both ends of femur are fixed with a four-hole dynamic compression plate. The diversion angle of two Steinman pins demonstrating external rotation of the distal fragment.

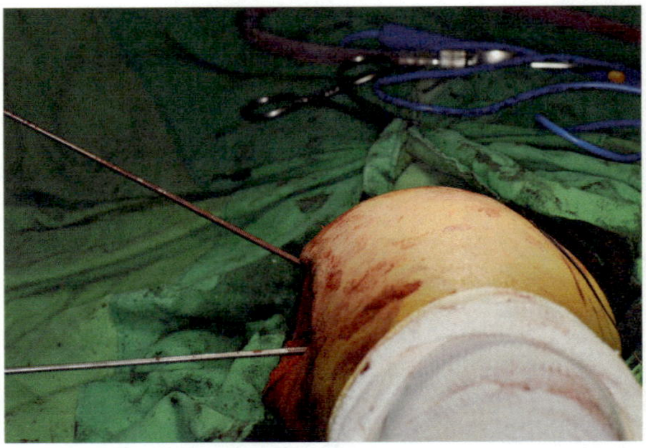

Figure 24. The diversion angle of two Steinmann pins viewing from caudally indicates the amount of external rotation (30° in this case) of the distal osteotomy.

http://dx.doi.org/10.5772/67516

6.8. Pitfalls and challenges

The Pemberton osteotomy is a well-established procedure and can be done safely by an experienced hand. The common complications included bleeding, infection, bone graft dislodgement, premature triradiate cartilage closure and re-dislocation. If the osteotomy is not stable enough to hold the bone graft, displacement of the graft may occur. If there is any doubt in the stability of the bone graft during operation, additional K-wire fixation for the osteotomy site through the bone graft should be done. Premature closure of the triradiate cartilage may develop if the osteotomy goes through the triradiate cartilage. But this complication is extremely rare. Re-dislocation of the hip after surgery is not a rare complication. The most common causes of re-dislocation are poor post-operative hip spica casting technique to hold the hip in reduced position, global deficiency of acetabulum, inexperienced surgeon and inadequate soft tissue release including iliopsoas tendon and transverse ligament. Excessive correction with Pemberton osteotomy may result in osteonecrosis of the femoral head and possibly femoral acetabular impingement in the future. Wu et al. have reported that with more distal femoral head positioning after pelvic osteotomy, there is a higher risk of osteonecrosis [6].

7. Long-term results

7.1. Change of hip joint anatomy

Concerns have been raised that redirection of the acetabulum with the Salter osteotomy may create an increased acetabular retroversion with improving anterior over-coverage. Acetabular retroversion or over anterior coverage has been implied as a cause of hip pain, impingement and subsequent osteoarthritis. In one study comparing long-term results of those two osteotomies, it suggested that by modifying the acetabular shape, the Pemberton osteotomy may result in an increase in anterior acetabular coverage. This in term may increase the risk of impingement [10]. Leg length discrepancy with longer leg at pathology side may be caused by coxa valga due to Kalamchi type II osteonecrosis of femoral head or trans-iliac lengthening of the pelvis [6].

7.2. Osteonecrosis of the femoral head

Osteonecrosis of the femoral head with physeal damage is not uncommon and a potentially devastating outcome following the treatment of DDH. The reported incidence of osteonecrosis has ranged from 0 to 73%. It is a severe complication that diminishes the long-term results of treatment of DDH. Although different treatment modalities have shown differences in the rates of osteonecrosis, most authors agree that an alteration of the blood supply to the femoral head resulting from treatment leads to this iatrogenic complication. It is generally accepted that the damaged blood supply of the proximal femoral epiphysis leads to osteonecrosis and the subsequent progressive deformity of the proximal femur [6]. The degree of osteonecrosis secondary to surgical treatment may range from mild epiphyseal hypoplasia to severe deformity of the femoral head depending on the location and extent of the physeal injury. Kalamchi and MacEwen's had developed four types of osteonecrosis after treatment of DDH [11]. Group I demonstrates changes affecting the ossific nucleus, group II is characterized by lateral physeal damage, group III has central physeal damage and group IV has total damage to the femoral head and physis. Patients with severe osteonecrosis (Kalamchi type III and IV) may lead to leg length discrepancy, joint incongruity and eventually premature OA. The majority (52%) of the cases of osteonecrosis after Pemberton osteotomy in the authors institute were Kalamchi type II with typical radiographic findings (coxa valga). Immobilization of a hip with an over-corrected acetabular fragment following osteotomy or immobilization of the hip in an extremely abducted position may compromise the blood supply of the proximal femoral epiphysis. It is believed that the lateral epiphyseal branch of the medial circumflex artery may be compressed by the acetabular labrum in the superior or the posterior intra-epiphyseal groove. Coxa valga due to Kalamchi type II osteonecrosis may not only lead to leg length discrepancy. Pelvic obliquity may also cause inadequate coverage of femoral head in the affected side. The decreased contact area between the femoral head and acetabulum may eventually lead to early osteoarthritis of hip. Wu et al. analysed long-term result of 167 patients who underwent Pemberton acetabuloplasty and found that excessive distal movement of the acetabular fragment was correlated with the development of osteonecrosis. They concluded that the risk of osteonecrosis is higher in those femoral head positioned more distally after Pemberton acetabuloplasty [6].

8. Treatment of long-term sequalae

Coxa valga caused by Kalamchi type II osteonecrosis of the femoral head can be treated by varus osteotomy of proximal femur or guided growth by an eccentric transphyseal screw. Leg length discrepancy can be treated by epiphysiodesis or modulation of the longer leg, or lengthening of the shorter limb by distraction osteogenesis.

9. Conclusion

For surgeons familiar with these procedures, either the Pemberton osteotomy or the Salter osteotomy can be a safe and effective option for treating developmental dysplasia of the hip. Careful surgical release of soft-tissue contractures, complete reduction, femoral shortening if indicated and avoidance of cast immobilization with the hip in an extreme position are believed to be effective in decreasing pressure on the femoral head and reducing the prevalence of osteonecrosis. Patients should be routinely followed until skeletal maturity to watch for long-term sequelae. Those treatable conditions should be appropriately managed at the right time to improve the long-term outcome.

Acknowledgements

Parts of this chapter are reproduced from Ref. [7].

Author details

Chunho Chen[1,2,3]*, Ting-Ming Wang[2,3] and Ken N. Kuo[2,3,4]

*Address all correspondence to: bacriv@gmail.com

1 Department of Orthopedic Surgery, Chiayi Christian Hospital, Chiayi, Taiwan

2 Department of Orthopedic Surgery, National Taiwan University Hospital, Taipei, Taiwan

3 School of Medicine, National Taiwan University, Taipei, Taiwan

4 Center for Evidence-Based Medicine, School of Medicine, Taipei Medical University, Taipei, Taiwan

References

[1] Pemberton PA. Pericapsular osteotomy of the ilium for treatment of congenital subluxation and dislocation of the hip. J Bone Joint Surg Am. 1965;47:65–86.

[2] Vedantam R, Capelli AM, Schoenecker PL. Pemberton osteotomy for the treatment of developmental dysplasia of the hip in older children. J Pediatr Orthop.1998;18:254–8.

[3] Wada A, Fujii T, Takamura K, Yanagida H, Taketa M, Nakamura T. Pemberton osteotomy for developmental dysplasia of the hip in older children. J Pediatr Orthop. 2003;23:508–13.

[4] Salter RB. Innominate osteotomy in the treatment of congenital dislocation and suluxation of the hip. J Bone Joint Surg Br. 1961;43:518–539.

[5] Salter RB and Dubos JP. The first fifteen-year personal experience with innominate osteotomy in the treatment of congenital dislocation and subluxation of the hip. Clin Orthop. 1974;98:72–103.

[6] Wu KW, Wang TM, Huang SC, Kuo KN, Chen CW. Analysis of osteonecrosis following Pemberton acetabuloplasty in deve-lopmental dysplasia of the hip: long-term results. J Bone Joint Surg Am. 2010;92:2083–94.

[7] Huang S-C, Wang T-M, Wu K-W, Fang C-F, Kuo KN. Pemberton osteotomy for acetabular dysplasia. JBJS Essential Surg Tech. 2011;94(1):1–1. DOI: 10.2106/JBJS.ST.K.00003

[8] Wang T-M, Wu K-W, Shih S-F, Huang S-C, Kuo KN. Outcomes of open reduction for developmental dysplasia of the hip: does bilateral dysplasia have a poorer outcome? J Bone Joint Surg Am. 2013;95(12):1081–6. DOI: 10.2106/JBJS.K.01324.

[9] Wang T-M, Wu K-W, Huang S-C, Huang W-C, Kuo KN. A Combined Procedure for High Dislocation in Patients with Developmental Dysplasia of the Hip. JBJS Essential Surg Tech. 2013;3(4):e19.

[10] Wang C-W, Wu K-W, Wang T-M, Huang S-C, Kuo KN. Comparison of acetabular anterior coverage after Salter osteotomy and Pemberton acetabuloplasty: a long-term followup. Clin Orthop Relat Res. 2014;472(3):1001–9. DOI: 10.1007/s11999-013-3319-6. Epub 2013 Oct 5.

[11] Kalamchi A, MacEwen GD. Avascular necrosis following treatment of congenital dislocation of the hip. J Bone Joint Surg Am. 1980;62:876–888.

Chapter 5

Total Hip Replacement in Developmental Dysplasia

Maximilian F. Kasparek and Friedrich Boettner

Additional information is available at the end of the chapter

http://dx.doi.org/10.5772/67480

Abstract

Total hip arthroplasty (THA) for osteoarthritis secondary to development dysplasia of the hip (DDH) is facing increasing levels of complexity with increasing grade of deformity. The dysplastic acetabulum is characterized by diminished bone stock with decreased lateral coverage. Therefore, it is challenging to restore the anatomic center of rotation and ensure adequate acetabular component fixation. Surgical strategies include a medialization of the acetabular component, a higher hip center, lateral structural bone grafting and the selection of smaller component sizes to improve native bone coverage. Excessive femoral anteversion is commonly encountered in patients with developmental dysplasia. Moreover, the intramedullary canal is narrow and the neck often aligned in valgus. Modular implants are helpful to address the altered femoral anatomy and also facilitate femoral shortening osteotomies in patients with high hip dislocation. Although clinical results are comparable to primary total hip replacement in primary osteoarthritis, the risk for revision surgery due to dislocation and loosening is increased. The current chapter reviews classification, preoperative planning, and surgical strategies for patients undergoing THA for osteoarthritis secondary to developmental dysplasia.

Keywords: developmental dysplasia, secondary osteoarthritis, primary total hip arthroplasty, bone grafting, femoral shortening osteotomy, complication

1. Introduction

Development dysplasia of the hip (DDH) is a common reason for primary total hip arthroplasty (THA) in young female adults. Surgical treatment is complicated by subluxation or dislocation of the femoral head out of the dysplastic acetabulum [1]. Complications occur more frequently due to the increased surgical complexity compared to THA in primary osteoarthritis. Understanding the underlying anatomical abnormalities in patients with DDH is of paramount importance for successful surgical treatment. The complexity is related to a dysplastic acetabulum with decreased lateral bone stock and coverage. Femoral anteversion is common especially in patients with lower levels of dysplasia [2]. In addition, most patients have a valgus neck alignment and a narrow medullary canal [3, 4].

2. Classification

The etiology of DDH is multifactorial and DDH is associated with positive family history and female gender [5]. Classification systems are based on the amount of displacement of the femoral head in relationship to the teardrop and predict the complexity of surgery. With increasing grade of deformity the acetabular bone stock is diminished. The most commonly used classification system was described by Crowe et al. [6] and Hartofilakidis et al. [7].

2.1. Crowe classification

Crowe et al. [6] classified DDH based on the grade of proximal subluxation of the femoral head (**Table 1**). The subluxation is calculated on anterior-posterior radiographs by measuring the proximal subluxation distance between the inter-teardrop line and the transition point of the femoral head to the femoral neck (**Figures 1** and **2**). The grade of subluxation is defined as the proximal subluxation in relation to the undeformed femoral head diameter.

In Crowe grade I, the proximal subluxation of the transition point is under <50% of the vertical femoral head diameter and in Crowe grade II between 50 and 74%. In grade III, proximal migration is about 75–100% and in grade IV more than 100% (**Table 1**).

If the femoral head is deformed, the vertical diameter of the femoral head is calculated as 20% of the height of the pelvis (distance between the iliac crest and the inferior margin of the ischial tuberosity).

The Crowe classification predicts the complexity of surgery and with increasing Crowe grade complications are more common [8]. Furthermore, it was reported that the Crowe classification correlates with grade of acetabular and femoral anteversion [2].

Grade	Crowe classification	Acetabular anteversion	Femoral anteversion
I	<50% subluxation	15°	42°
II	50–74% subluxation	10°	30°
III	75–100% subluxation	7°	43°
IV	>100% subluxation	4°	27°

Table 1. Crowe classification and relationship with acetabular and femoral anteversion [2, 6].

http://dx.doi.org/10.5772/67480

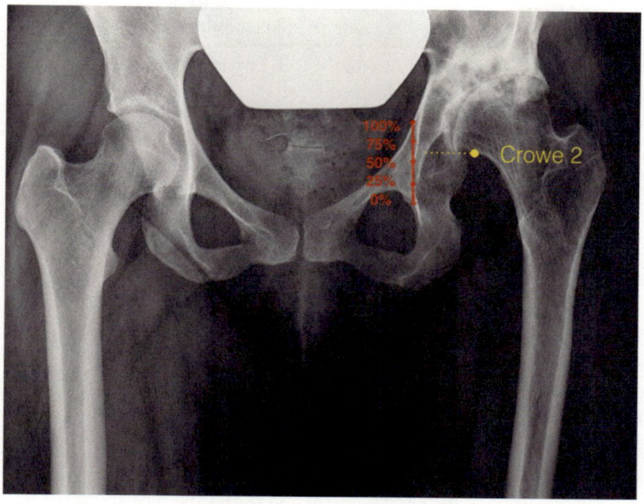

Figure 1. On the radiographs a Crowe grade II deformity is shown (50–74% subluxation). The subluxation is calculated by measuring the proximal migration between the teardrop line and the transition point of femoral head-neck.

2.2. Hartofilakidis classification

Hartofilakidis et al. [7] classified dysplastic hips in three overall categories based on radiographic appearance of the hip: in Type A the femoral head is articulating with the true acetabulum; in Type B the femoral head articulate with a false acetabulum and the false and true acetabulum are still connected; finally in a Type C the femoral head has migrated further proximal (**Table 2**) and therefore true and actual acetabulum are separated. This classification

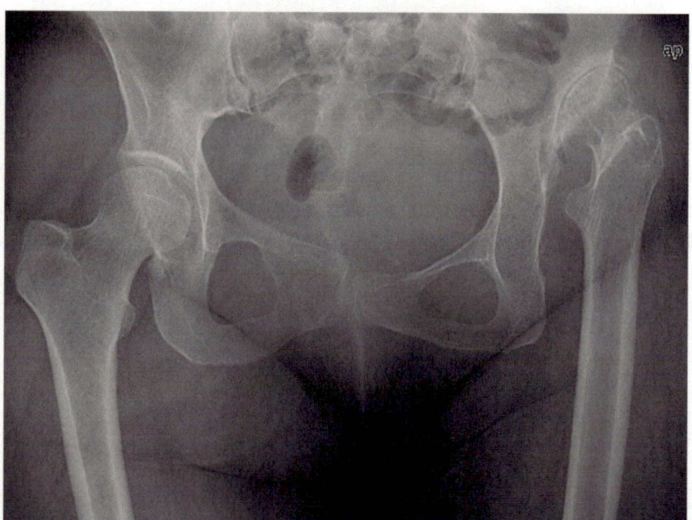

Figure 2. Radiograph of a Crowe grade IV deformity.

Hartofilakidis		Acetabular deficiency
Type A	The femoral head is contained within the original acetabulum despite some degree of subluxation	1. Superior segmental deficiency 2. Secondary shallowing due to fossa-covering osteophyte
Type B	The femoral head articulates with a false acetabulum that partially covers the true acetabulum	1. Anterior and posterior segmental deficiency 2. Narrow opening 3. Inadequate depth 4. Increased anteversion
Type C	With high dislocation, the femoral head has migrated superiorly and posteriorly. The true acetabulum is inferior and anterior to the false acetabulum along the iliac wing	1. Segmental deficiency of the entire acetabular rim 2. Narrow opening 3. Inadequate depth 4. Excessive anteversion 5. Abnormal distribution of bone stock, mainly superoposteriorly

Table 2. Hartofilakidis classification [7].

system describes the anatomical deformity and predicts the complexity of acetabular reconstruction.

3. Preoperative planning

Standardized radiographs including calibrated anterior-posterior (AP) pelvis radiographs at the level of the anterior superior iliac spine and lateral hip views are required for templating. Standard AP pelvis radiographs including the iliac crest are necessary to grade the DDH using the Crowe classification. Computer tomography is useful for determining: (1) acetabular component position and bone stock, (2) the amount of femoral anteversion, and (3) the size of the femoral canal in order to determine if standard implants are feasible. Preoperative planning should incorporate planning of the center of rotation before and after surgery as well as the need for femoral shortening osteotomies. This is essential to restore adequate leg lengths. In addition, overall amount of lengthening should be determined to anticipate the risk of sciatic nerve palsy. Adequate sizing of the femoral canal is important in patients at risk for a shortening osteotomy (Crowe type 3 and 4) to assure adequate distal press fit.

4. Surgical approaches

Surgeons should use the surgical approach they are most comfortable with. Standard surgical approaches include the direct anterior, anterolateral, direct lateral, and posterior

http://dx.doi.org/10.5772/67480

approach. Advantages of the lateral and posterior approaches are a good view of the acetabulum. The posterior approach also facilitates the access to the femur for shortening osteotomies. While the posterior approach has advantages for patients with more deficient lateral bone stock and high hip dislocations, the direct anterior approach facilitates acetabular component reaming and placement due to intraoperative C-Arm imaging [9]. In addition, operating in a supine position facilitates restoration of leg length. Moreover, in cases with prior periacetabular osteotomies the surgeon can often utilize the same incision [10].

In patients with severe DDH that require shortening osteotomy, it is advantageous to start with femoral preparation since the shortening osteotomy itself often greatly facilitates acetabular exposure. Occasionally, a sliding trochanteric osteotomy can be required to improve abductor muscle tension [11]. Also the posterior capsule and external rotators should be preserved and repaired to reduce the risk of postoperative dislocation [12]. Postoperative weight bearing status is influenced by the type of surgical reconstruction and implant rather than the surgical approach. More advanced postoperative precautions are usually applied to patients undergoing a posterior and direct lateral approach.

5. Acetabular component implantation

In DDH, the acetabulum is often shallow and oval. This results in altered anatomic landmarks and it can be challenging to identify the true acetabulum. Identifying the teardrop (junction of the ischium and pubis) either clinically or using intraoperative fluoroscopy is of absolute importance to locate the true acetabulum [13].

Finding the balance between restoration of the center of rotation and adequate lateral bone coverage requires careful preoperative templating and surgical experience. Lateral coverage can be improved by medialization of the cup and decreasing its size to improve coverage in case of lateral bone deficiency.

In most cases the center of rotation is slightly elevated to improve lateral coverage. This does impact on postoperative leg length and needs to be carefully considered when restoring postoperative leg lengths. Finding the right compromise is also important to avoid a high hip center that can affect postoperative function [1, 14, 15]. In addition, a high hip center increases the forces on the acetabulum and can increase the risk for cup loosening [16, 17]. Therefore, in general it is recommended to restore the center of rotation within 15 mm of the center of the true acetabulum or <35 mm superior to the interteardrop line [18].

A modern porous coated spherical cup, including smaller sizes (40–46 mm) should be available with maximal head size to improve stability. During acetabular reaming, the anterior wall should be protected, as it is often very thin and most of the bone stock is available posterior (**Figure 3**). Therefore, the authors recommend to ream preferentially

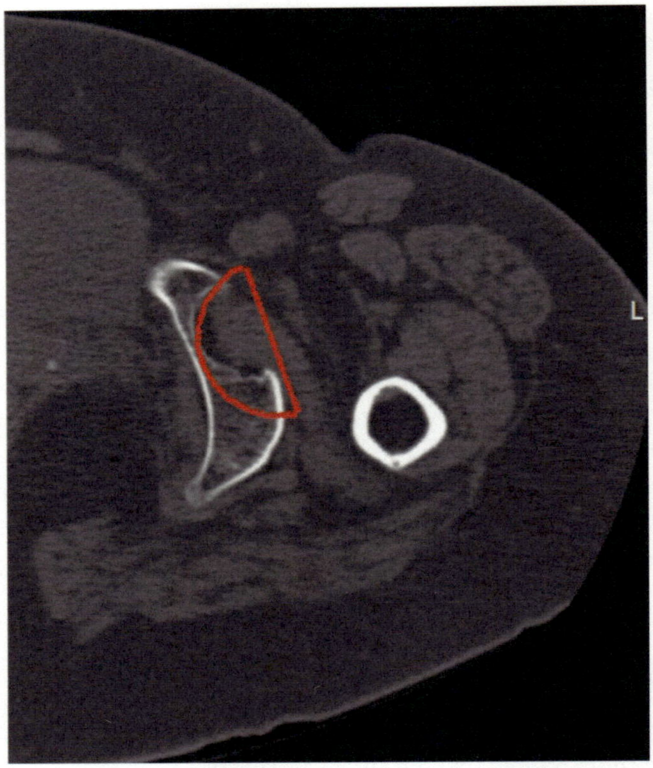

Figure 3. Computer tomography reveals that in the posterior part of the acetabulum there is more bone stock available. Reaming should be done more posteriorly to protect the anterior wall of the acetabulum.

posterior. While medialization is important, care should be taken to avoid over medialization with loss of medial bone fixation. The authors prefer reaching the inner table without penetrating it completely. Whenever the cup extends medially beyond Kohler's line medial bone grafting with graft from the reamer can help later restoration of the medial wall.

Lack of lateral coverage up to 17 mm of uncovered implant arc is acceptable for all implant sizes [19]. For larger acetabular components (52 and up) with less than 45 degree of cup inclination up to 25 mm of the cup can remain uncovered. If preoperative templating suggests that a larger area of the cup is not covered by bone than lateral bone grafting, utilizing the femoral head fixed with two screws (Harris plastic) is recommended [20] (**Figure 4**). Good long-term results with incorporation of the graft were reported for this technique [21, 22]. Metal augments can alternatively be utilized to improve lateral fixation [23], however, the authors prefer a biological restoration of bone stock using the Harris plastic. To facilitate the graft fixation and reaming, it is usually advised to make the decision to proceed with bone grafting early during the acetabular reaming. Modern robotic cup implantation using the Mako® system (Stryker, Kalamazoo, MI) allows for perfect reaming of the acetabulum

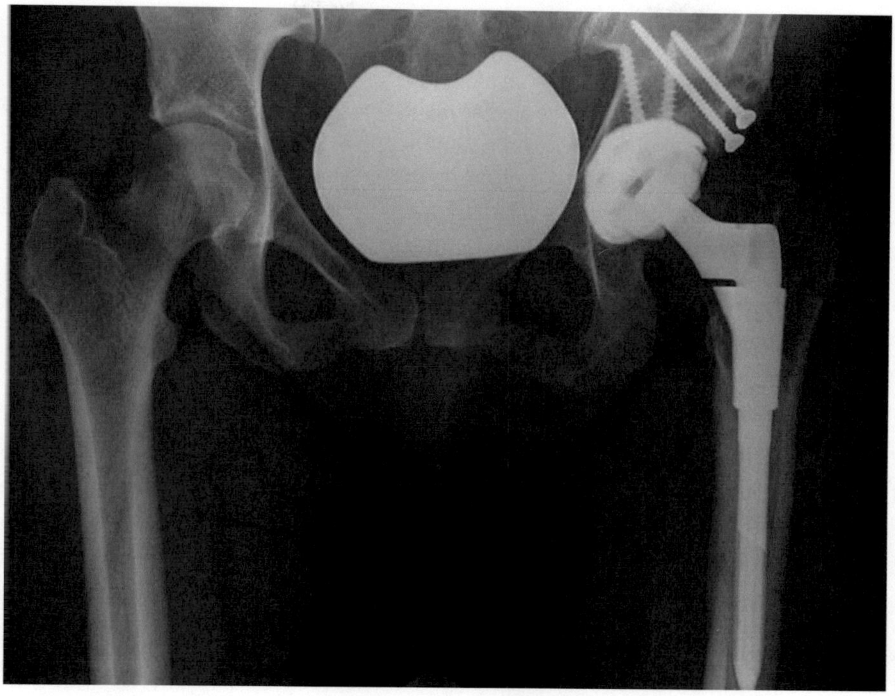

Figure 4. Postoperative radiographs after restoration of a Crowe grade III deformity. The anatomical hip center is restored with a femoral bone graft (Harris plastic).

according to the preoperative plan and is an appealing treatment option for patients undergoing THA for DDH.

5.1. Crowe classification: how it impacts acetabular fixation

In Crowe grade 1 deformities acetabular component fixation is often not too difficult, because in most cases adequate bone stock is available. Therefore, good implant-bone coverage can be achieved almost always without bone grafting or excessive medialization.

Crowe grade II and III deformities are the most difficult defects to restore. In these deformities the femoral head is more subluxated, and significant parts of the lateral bone stock are missing. However, while most Crowe 2 and 3 can be managed similar to grade I by placing the cup proximal-medial and by using a smaller cup size, occasionally a Harris plastic is indicated.

Crowe grade IV deformities are easier to manage because the femoral head was dislocated from the acetabulum without continuous pressure on the lateral bone stock. In most cases the hip center can be restored with a smaller acetabular component in anatomic position. In these cases care should be taken not to over ream since the bone is often soft due to the lack of weight bearing. Restoration of the center of rotation in Crowe grade IV might require a femoral shortening osteotomy to facilitate reduction of the hip.

6. Femoral reconstruction

In comparison to patients with primary osteoarthritis, the dysplastic femur has a narrower and straighter intramedullary canal [24, 25]. In mildly dysplastic hips standard femoral stems can often be used. However, the proximal bone is often osteopenic and its valgus alignment can increase the risk of calcar fractures if broached implants are used. A femoral wire-cerclage of the proximal femur just above the lesser trochanter can be used prophylactically.

Modular implants (for instance S-Rom® system, DePuy, Warsaw, IN) allow the surgeon to use a standard implant for patients with small canal diameter and excessive anteversion while preserving the option to do a femoral shortening osteotomy [26]. The proximal modular sleeve can be selected according to the proximal metaphysis shape and size.

Modular implants also allow to correct excessive anteversion and adjusts the medial spout according to the amount of valgus present [12]. Surgeons should be aware that excessive femoral anteversion is more common in patients with lower Crowe grades. Excessive femoral anteversion can also be corrected using derotation of the proximal fragment during a femoral shortening osteotomy [13].

In grade Crowe III and especially IV, subtrochanteric shortening osteotomies are often indicated [27]. Limb lengthening is generally possible between 2.5 and 4.5 cm [28]. If more lengthening is required, femoral shortening is recommended to avoid sciatic nerve palsy [29, 30]. Especially patients with prior surgeries are at increased risk for sciatic nerve palsy and less lengthening might be possible in these patients.

Preoperative planning is crucial to assess the location of the osteotomy, diameter of the stem as well as extend of lengthening. While a shortening osteotomy can be performed using a cemented stem, today, usually a modular uncemented femoral component is preferred. The removed bone segment can be split in coronal plane and utilized as bone graft by wiring the bone shells on each side of the osteotomy to improve rotational stability. Theoretically, an oblique osteotomy can improve rotational stability; today transverse osteotomies are usually preferred to facilitate derotation of the proximal fragment.

Alternatives to shortening osteotomies are swan neck prosthesis or two stage skeletal traction followed by THA [31–33].

To facilitate intraoperative reduction soft tissue releases including release of the gluteus maximus insertion on the proximal femur, elevation of the gluteus medius of its insertion on the ilium, release of the psoas off the lesser trochanter as well as releases of the anterior and posterior capsule might be necessary. In case of a severe adduction contracture, a postoperative percutaneous release of the adductor tendons can be considered. It is crucial to carefully balance the need for soft tissue releases to facilitate reduction and the need for stability of the hip to minimize postoperative dislocations.

Recommended bearing options in THA for DDH are metal or ceramic on highly crosslinked polyethylene-bearing combinations.

7. Hip resurfacing

In young male patients with Crowe grade I or II deformity, hip resurfacing can be a valuable treatment option with satisfactory results [34, 35]. However, hip resurfacing can face a number of challenges in patients with DDH: because of the valgus neck alignment restoration of hip offset is usually challenging; excessive femoral anteversion and leg shortening cannot be corrected using a hip resurfacing; finally, acetabular components rely on primary press fit and screw augmentation is not possible for most resurfacing components. If a limb-length discrepancy of more than 2 cm or a Crowe grade III or IV deformity is present, hip resurfacing is not recommended [36]. Advantages of hip resurfacing include preservation of bone stock, better range of motion, and stability as well as increased ability to participate in sport compared to conventional THA.

8. Postoperative mobilization

While early mobilization is encouraged in patients undergoing THA for DDH, patients requiring modular implants or more advanced bone grafting and shortening osteotomies often need to observe toe touch weight bearing on crutches for 4–6 weeks. Standard postoperative antithrombotic prophylaxis is recommended.

Shortening osteotomies might require additional abductor precautions during the first 4–6 weeks. Hip precautions are usually enforced for patients undergoing a posterior approach.

9. Complications

Complications are more common in patients undergoing THA for DDH [37]. A higher incidence of proximal femoral fractures is encountered due to the dysplastic narrow femoral canal.

The incidence of dislocations in dysplastic hips is increased and postoperative dislocation is the most common reason for revision surgeries within the first 6 months [38]. Dislocations are commonly anterior as a result of extensive combined anteversion and are not influenced by Crowe grade or the need for shortening osteotomies [39]. Moreover, smaller head diameters due to smaller acetabular component sizes and a decreased femoral offset are additional risk factors for dislocation. The medialization of the cup can result in a decreased femoral offset and bony impingement.

Increased polyethylene wear can occur because of the smaller component sizes with thinner polyethylene inserts, resulting in osteolysis and acetabular component loosening [40].

Also the risk for sciatic nerve palsy is increased and its risk is associated with surgical complexity and history of prior surgeries [41]. Nonunion or delayed union can be encountered in patients with femoral shortening osteotomies [42, 43].

A higher incidence of infections was reported for patients undergoing THA for DDH compared to osteoarthritis. This might be secondary to the increased surgical complexity, increased surgical time, as well as the need for extensive soft tissue releases and utilization of bone grafts [13].

10. Outcome

The functional outcome of THA in DDH is comparable to primary THA in osteoarthritis [44, 45]. However, the revision rate is higher compared to patients with osteoarthritis and increases with severity of the deformity [8, 37]. Increased revision rates in cemented components due to loosening and increased wear were reported in the past, but modern implants and surgical techniques have remarkably improved the long-term survival rates [46]. Even in cases with shortening osteotomies modern implants provide satisfactory mid- and long-term functional results [47, 48].

A proper restoration of hip mechanics and soft tissue balance is important to provide the best functional results after THA. An anatomical restoration of the hip center improves function and decreases acetabular component loosening [18]. Functional results in severe DDH are poor compared to primary osteoarthritis [42], which might be related to the accompanying soft tissue contractures and preoperative functional status. Patients may also have a limb after surgery due to muscle weakness of the abductors. However, in general THA in DDH provides significant increase in function and quality of life in the long-term follow up [49]. Prior pelvis osteotomies can increase the surgical complexity, but do not influence the complication rate or outcome [50, 51].

11. Conclusion

Preoperative planning is crucial in developmental dysplasia. With increasing grade of deformity, the surgeon should have special modular implants available and should be prepared to perform femoral shortening osteotomies as well as lateral acetabular bone grafting. Modern THA provides good long-term results, however, complication rates are increased compared to THA in primary osteoarthritis. It is important to communicate realistic expectations, discuss the increased risk of complications and alert the patient to the possible need for protected weight-bearing.

Contribution statement

I attest to the fact that all authors have participated in the research, read the manuscript, attest to the validity and legitimacy of the data and its interpretation, and agree to its submission.

Conflict of interest statement

We certify that we have not signed any agreement with commercial interest related to this book chapter, which would in any way limit publication of any and all data generated for the study or to delay publication for any reason.

Dr. Boettner reports personal fees from Smith & Nephew, personal fees from Ortho Development Corporation and personal fees form DePuy, outside the submitted work.

Author details

Maximilian F. Kasparek and Friedrich Boettner*

*Address all correspondence to: boettnerf@hss.edu

Adult Reconstruction and Joint Replacement Division, Hospital for Special Surgery, New York, NY, USA

References

[1] Hartofilakidis G, Karachalios T. Total hip arthroplasty for congenital hip disease. J Bone Joint Surg Am 2004;86-a(2):242–50.

[2] Bernasek TL, Haidukewych GJ, Gustke KA, Hill O, Levering M. Total hip arthroplasty requiring subtrochanteric osteotomy for developmental hip dysplasia: 5- to 14-year results. J Arthroplasty 2007;22(6 Suppl 2):145–50. doi:10.1016/j.arth.2007.05.014.

[3] Argenson JN, Flecher X, Parratte S, Aubaniac JM. Anatomy of the dysplastic hip and consequences for total hip arthroplasty. Clin Orthop Relat Res 2007;465:40–5. doi:10.1097/BLO.0b013e3181576052.

[4] Argenson JN, Ryembault E, Flecher X, Brassart N, Parratte S, Aubaniac JM. Three-dimensional anatomy of the hip in osteoarthritis after developmental dysplasia. J Bone Joint Surg Br 2005;87(9):1192–6. doi:10.1302/0301-620x.87b9.15928.

[5] Hoaglund FT, Shiba R, Newberg AH, Leung KY. Diseases of the hip. A comparative study of Japanese Oriental and American white patients. J Bone Joint Surg Am 1985; 67(9):1376–83.

[6] Crowe JF, Mani VJ, Ranawat CS. Total hip replacement in congenital dislocation and dysplasia of the hip. J Bone Joint Surg Am 1979;61(1):15–23.

[7] Hartofilakidis G, Stamos K, Karachalios T, Ioannidis TT, Zacharakis N. Congenital hip disease in adults. Classification of acetabular deficiencies and operative treat-

ment with acetabuloplasty combined with total hip arthroplasty. J Bone Joint Surg Am 1996;78(5):683–92.

[8] Cameron HU, Botsford DJ, Park YS. Influence of the Crowe rating on the outcome of total hip arthroplasty in congenital hip dysplasia. J Arthroplasty 1996;11(5):582–7.

[9] Gromov K, Greene ME, Huddleston JI, Emerson R, Gebuhr P, Malchau H et al. Acetabular dysplasia and surgical approaches other than direct anterior increases risk for malpositioning of the acetabular component in total hip arthroplasty. J Arthroplasty 2016;31(4):835–41. doi:10.1016/j.arth.2015.10.045.

[10] Baque F, Brown A, Matta J. Total hip arthroplasty after periacetabular osteotomy. Orthopedics 2009;32(6):399. doi:10.3928/01477447-20090511-04.

[11] Lakstein D, Backstein DJ, Safir O, Kosashvili Y, Gross AE. Modified trochanteric slide for complex hip arthroplasty: clinical outcomes and complication rates. J Arthroplasty 2010;25(3):363–8. doi:10.1016/j.arth.2009.02.017.

[12] Sanchez-Sotelo J, Berry DJ, Trousdale RT, Cabanela ME. Surgical treatment of developmental dysplasia of the hip in adults: II. Arthroplasty options. J Am Acad Orthop Surg 2002;10(5):334–44.

[13] Rogers BA, Garbedian S, Kuchinad RA, Backstein D, Safir O, Gross AE. Total hip arthroplasty for adult hip dysplasia. J Bone Joint Surg Am 2012;94(19):1809–21. doi:10.2106/jbjs.k.00779.

[14] Doehring TC, Rubash HE, Shelley FJ, Schwendeman LJ, Donaldson TK, Navalgund YA. Effect of superior and superolateral relocations of the hip center on hip joint forces. An experimental and analytical analysis. J Arthroplasty 1996;11(6):693–703.

[15] Delp SL, Wixson RL, Komattu AV, Kocmond JH. How superior placement of the joint center in hip arthroplasty affects the abductor muscles. Clin Orthop Relat Res 1996;(328):137–46.

[16] Bicanic G, Delimar D, Delimar M, Pecina M. Influence of the acetabular cup position on hip load during arthroplasty in hip dysplasia. Int Orthop 2009;33(2):397–402. doi:10.1007/s00264-008-0683-z.

[17] Stans AA, Pagnano MW, Shaughnessy WJ, Hanssen AD. Results of total hip arthroplasty for Crowe Type III developmental hip dysplasia. Clin Orthop Relat Res 1998;(348): 149–57.

[18] Watts CD, Abdel MP, Hanssen AD, Pagnano MW. Anatomic hip center decreases aseptic loosening rates after total hip arthroplasty with cement in patients with Crowe type-II dysplasia: a concise follow-up report at a mean of thirty-six years. J Bone Joint Surg Am 2016;98(11):910–5. doi:10.2106/jbjs.15.00902.

[19] Li H, Mao Y, Oni JK, Dai K, Zhu Z. Total hip replacement for developmental dysplasia of the hip with more than 30% lateral uncoverage of uncemented acetabular components. Bone Joint J 2013;95-b(9):1178–83. doi:10.1302/0301-620x.95b9.31398.

[20] Harris WH, Crothers O, Oh I. Total hip replacement and femoral-head bone-grafting for severe acetabular deficiency in adults. J Bone Joint Surg Am 1977;59(6):752–9.

[21] Spangehl MJ, Berry DJ, Trousdale RT, Cabanela ME. Uncemented acetabular components with bulk femoral head autograft for acetabular reconstruction in developmental dysplasia of the hip: results at five to twelve years. J Bone Joint Surg Am 2001;83-a(10):1484–9.

[22] Abdel MP, Stryker LS, Trousdale RT, Berry DJ, Cabanela ME. Uncemented acetabular components with femoral head autograft for acetabular reconstruction in developmental dysplasia of the hip: a concise follow-up report at a mean of twenty years. J Bone Joint Surg Am 2014;96(22):1878–82. doi:10.2106/jbjs.n.00061.

[23] Bicanic G, Barbaric K, Bohacek I, Aljinovic A, Delimar D. Current concept in dysplastic hip arthroplasty: techniques for acetabular and femoral reconstruction. World J Orthop 2014;5(4):412–24. doi:10.5312/wjo.v5.i4.412.

[24] Noble PC, Kamaric E, Sugano N, Matsubara M, Harada Y, Ohzono K et al. Three-dimensional shape of the dysplastic femur: implications for THR. Clin Orthop Relat Res 2003;(417):27–40. doi:30.3097/01.blo.0000096819.67494.32.

[25] Robertson DD, Essinger JR, Imura S, Kuroki Y, Sakamaki T, Shimizu T et al. Femoral deformity in adults with developmental hip dysplasia. Clin Orthop Relat Res 1996;(327):196–206.

[26] Tamegai H, Otani T, Fujii H, Kawaguchi Y, Hayama T, Marumo K. A modified S-ROM stem in primary total hip arthroplasty for developmental dysplasia of the hip. J Arthroplasty 2013;28(10):1741–5. doi:10.1016/j.arth.2013.04.041.

[27] Gustke K. The dysplastic hip: not for the shallow surgeon. Bone Joint J 2013;95-b(11 Suppl A):31–6. doi:10.1302/0301-620x.95b11.32899.

[28] Lewallen DG. Neurovascular injury associated with hip arthroplasty. Instr Course Lect 1998;47:275–83.

[29] Sener N, Tozun IR, Asik M. Femoral shortening and cementless arthroplasty in high congenital dislocation of the hip. J Arthroplasty 2002;17(1):41–8.

[30] Reikeraas O, Lereim P, Gabor I, Gunderson R, Bjerkreim I. Femoral shortening in total arthroplasty for completely dislocated hips: 3–7 year results in 25 cases. Acta Orthop Scand 1996;67(1):33–6.

[31] Huo MH, Salvati EA, Lieberman JR, Burstein AH, Wilson PD, Jr. Custom-designed femoral prostheses in total hip arthroplasty done with cement for severe dysplasia of the hip. J Bone Joint Surg Am 1993;75(10):1497–504.

[32] DiFazio F, Shon WY, Salvati EA, Wilson PD, Jr. Long-term results of total hip arthroplasty with a cemented custom-designed swan-neck femoral component for congenital dislocation or severe dysplasia: a follow-up note. J Bone Joint Surg Am 2002;84-a(2):204–7.

[33] Yoon PW, Kim JI, Kim DO, Yu CH, Yoo JJ, Kim HJ et al. Cementless total hip arthroplasty for patients with Crowe type III or IV developmental dysplasia of the hip: two-stage total hip arthroplasty following skeletal traction after soft tissue release for irreducible hips. Clin Orthop Surg 2013;5(3):167–73. doi:10.4055/cios.2013.5.3.167.

[34] Wang Q, Zhang XL, Chen YS, Shen H, Shao JJ. Resurfacing arthroplasty for hip dysplasia: a prospective randomised study. J Bone Joint Surg Br 2012;94(6):768–73. doi:10.1302/0301-620x.94b6.28522.

[35] Amstutz HC, Le Duff MJ, Harvey N, Hoberg M. Improved survivorship of hybrid metal-on-metal hip resurfacing with second-generation techniques for Crowe-I and II developmental dysplasia of the hip. J Bone Joint Surg Am 2008;90 Suppl 3:12–20. doi:10.2106/jbjs.h.00711.

[36] Amstutz HC, Beaule PE, Dorey FJ, Le Duff MJ, Campbell PA, Gruen TA. Metal-on-metal hybrid surface arthroplasty. Surgical Technique. J Bone Joint Surg Am 2006;88 Suppl 1 Pt 2:234–49. doi:10.2106/jbjs.f.00273.

[37] Krych AJ, Howard JL, Trousdale RT, Cabanela ME, Berry DJ. Total hip arthroplasty with shortening subtrochanteric osteotomy in Crowe type-IV developmental dysplasia. J Bone Joint Surg Am 2009;91(9):2213–21. doi:10.2106/jbjs.h.01024.

[38] Thillemann TM, Pedersen AB, Johnsen SP, Soballe K. Implant survival after primary total hip arthroplasty due to childhood hip disorders: results from the Danish Hip Arthroplasty Registry. Acta Orthop 2008;79(6):769–76. doi:10.1080/17453670810016830.

[39] Wang L, Trousdale RT, Ai S, An KN, Dai K, Morrey BF. Dislocation after total hip arthroplasty among patients with developmental dysplasia of the hip. J Arthroplasty 2012;27(5):764–9. doi:10.1016/j.arth.2011.08.021.

[40] Murray PJ, Hwang KL, Imrie SN, Huddleston JI, 3rd, Goodman SB. Polyethylene wear and osteolysis is associated with high revision rate of a small sized porous coated THA in patients with hip dysplasia. J Arthroplasty 2014;29(7):1373–7. doi:10.1016/j.arth.2014.02.027.

[41] Eggli S, Hankemayer S, Muller ME. Nerve palsy after leg lengthening in total replacement arthroplasty for developmental dysplasia of the hip. J Bone Joint Surg Br 1999;81(5):843–5.

[42] Yalcin N, Kilicarslan K, Karatas F, Mutlu T, Yildirim H. Cementless total hip arthroplasty with subtrochanteric transverse shortening osteotomy for severely dysplastic or dislocated hips. Hip Int 2010;20(1):87–93.

[43] Hartofilakidis G, Babis GC, Georgiades G, Kourlaba G. Trochanteric osteotomy in total hip replacement for congenital hip disease. J Bone Joint Surg Br 2011;93(5):601–7. doi:10.1302/0301-620x.93b5.24780.

[44] Boyle MJ, Frampton CM, Crawford HA. Early results of total hip arthroplasty in patients with developmental dysplasia of the hip compared with patients with osteoarthritis. J Arthroplasty 2012;27(3):386–90. doi:10.1016/j.arth.2011.06.024.

[45] Engesaeter LB, Furnes O, Havelin LI. Developmental dysplasia of the hip—good results of later total hip arthroplasty: 7135 primary total hip arthroplasties after developmental dysplasia of the hip compared with 59774 total hip arthroplasties in idiopathic coxarthrosis followed for 0 to 15 years in the Norwegian Arthroplasty Register. J Arthroplasty 2008;23(2):235–40. doi:10.1016/j.arth.2007.03.023.

[46] Perka C, Fischer U, Taylor WR, Matziolis G. Developmental hip dysplasia treated with total hip arthroplasty with a straight stem and a threaded cup. J Bone Joint Surg Am 2004;86-a(2):312–9.

[47] Takao M, Ohzono K, Nishii T, Miki H, Nakamura N, Sugano N. Cementless modular total hip arthroplasty with subtrochanteric shortening osteotomy for hips with developmental dysplasia. J Bone Joint Surg Am 2011;93(6):548–55. doi:10.2106/jbjs.i.01619.

[48] Park MS, Kim KH, Jeong WC. Transverse subtrochanteric shortening osteotomy in primary total hip arthroplasty for patients with severe hip developmental dysplasia. J Arthroplasty 2007;22(7):1031–6. doi:10.1016/j.arth.2007.05.011.

[49] Roidis NT, Pollalis AP, Hartofilakidis GC. Total hip arthroplasty in young females with congenital dislocation of the hip, radically improves their long-term quality of life. J Arthroplasty 2013;28(7):1206–11. doi:10.1016/j.arth.2012.09.025.

[50] Tokunaga K, Aslam N, Zdero R, Schemitsch EH, Waddell JP. Effect of prior Salter or Chiari osteotomy on THA with developmental hip dysplasia. Clin Orthop Relat Res 2011;469(1):237–43. doi:10.1007/s11999-010-1375-8.

[51] Duncan S, Wingerter S, Keith A, Fowler SA, Clohisy J. Does previous osteotomy compromise total hip arthroplasty? A systematic review. J Arthroplasty 2015;30(1):79–85. doi:10.1016/j.arth.2014.08.030.

Chapter 6

Total Hip Replacement in Developmental Dysplasia of the Hip: Pitfalls and Challenges

Özgür Korkmaz and Melih Malkoç

Additional information is available at the end of the chapter

http://dx.doi.org/10.5772/67479

Abstract

Introduction: Surgical treatment methods for developmental dysplasia of the hip (DDH) in the elderly patients contain pelvic or periacetabular osteotomy and hip arthroplasty. Total hip arthroplasty (THA) is the last and definitive surgical treatment modality for the end stage developmental dysplasia of the hip.

Deformity classification and reconstruction: Crowe classification system describes the degree of dysplasia and gives information about the reconstruction procedure with hip arthroplasty. Classification is based on the magnitude of proximal femoral migration relative to the acetabulum. Acetabular component must be implanted to the true acetabulum for the optimal range of motion and stability of the reconstructed hip. The femoral component must be placed in neutral or slight anteversion but narrow femoral canal can be a problem for the reconstruction of femur.

Conclusion—key results: The results of total hip arthroplasty in developmental dysplasia of the hip have been satisfactory for stability, mobility, and pain relief. The survivorship of cemented arthroplasty in dysplastic hips is inferior because of the young age of the patients and the complexity of the procedures. Early and midterm results of cementless hip arthroplasty are better. Most important complications after the surgery are dislocation of the reconstructed hip and sciatic nerve injury.

Keywords: hip, arthroplasty, developmental dysplasia

1. Introduction

Hip arthroplasty is the end stage treatment method for developmental dysplasia of the hip (DDH). Pelvic and femoral osteotomies are the first option for surgical treatment. Before performing osteotomies, cartilage space in the hip joint must be determined. It must be verified with X-rays. In the long-term follow-up after pelvic or femoral osteotomies, degenerative changes occur in the hip joint. Also, hip arthroplasty is the last stage treatment modality after osteotomies around hip joint.

Hip arthroplasty for developmental dysplasia of the hip is technically complex surgical procedure because of the anatomical changes of acetabulum and proximal part of the femur. Soft tissue contractures and laxity can be present as a result of the acetabular and proximal femoral anatomical differences.

Patients with dysplasia require arthroplasty in younger age than the others with osteoarthritis. For this reason, implant selection is an important issue. Bearing surfaces alternative to metal on polyethylene should be preferred in this young patient population.

2. Anatomical differences in developmental dysplasia of the hip

2.1. Acetabular abnormalities

An acetabulum with dysplasia can be shallow, narrow, and lateralized. Increased anteversion and deficiency of the anterior and superior walls of acetabulum are changes expected to be seen in these patients [1]. The width of acetabulum remains same, but there is an increase in length and decrease in depth [2, 3]. As a result of these deformities, the coverage of the femoral head by the acetabulum has deficiency anteriorly, laterally, and superiorly. Completely dislocated hips have a false acetabulum on ilium with joint capsule. True acetabulum is hypoplastic and invaded with adipose tissue.

2.2. Femoral abnormalities

The dysplastic femur has a small femoral head. Femoral neck anteversion has increased. Generally, femoral neck is shortened with an increased neck-shaft angle [3]. There can be posterior displacement of trochanter major and a narrow femoral canal can be seen [1]. Narrowing of medullary canal around the level of the lesser trochanter is evident in Crowe IV DDH [4].

2.3. Soft tissue abnormalities

The abductor muscles orientation becomes transverse. Hypertrophies can be seen in psoas tendon and hip capsule. The hamstrings, adductors, and rectus femoris muscles shorten. Also, ligamentum teres and labral hypertrophies occur. For patients with unilateral DDH, the sciatic nerve lies close to the ischium and ilium but far from the femur of DDH when compared to healthy side. Sciatic nerve becomes shorter in the affected side, and it can be injured by posterolateral approach [5].

3. Classification of developmental dysplasia of the hip

There are several classification systems for developmental dysplasia of hip. Most popular ones are that were defined by Crowe and Hartofilakidis [6, 7]. There are three grades according to Hartofilakidis classification. The femoral head is covered within the true acetabulum in the first grade. In the second grade, femoral head has an articulation with the false acetabulum, and there is a contact between inferior lip of the false acetabulum and superior lip of the true acetabulum. This type is also called low dislocation. In the third grade, the femoral head is outside the true or the false acetabulum, and there is no articulation between femoral head and acetabulum. It is called high dislocation [7].

Crowe classification is a radiological classification based on proximal migration of the femoral head. There are four categories in this classification. The migration is calculated by measuring the vertical distance between the inter-teardrop line and the medial head-neck junction of hip. The stage of the subluxation is determined by the ratio of this distance to the vertical diameter of the opposite femoral head. If this ratio is less than 50% type 1, between 50% and 75% type II, between 75% and 100% type III, and greater than 100% subluxation type IV [6] (**Figure 1**).

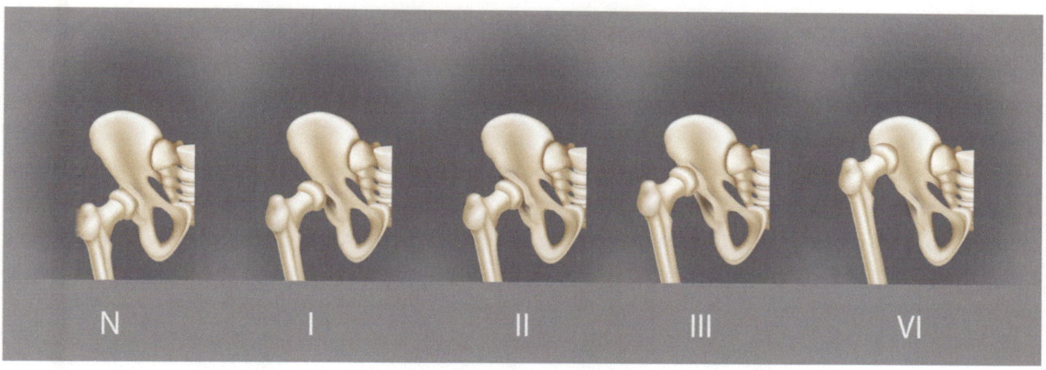

Figure 1. Crowe classification for developmental dysplasia of the hip.

4. Preoperative evaluation

Total hip arthroplasty (THA) is recommended for patients with end-stage disease who have pain and restriction in activities of daily living. Hip range of motion must be evaluated. Limb length inequality of the effected extremity must be measured. Anteroposterior views of the pelvis and hip radiographs should be taken. Lateral views of the hip and Judet views can be helpful to determine the acetabular bone stock. CT scan can be useful to evaluate acetabular bone stock and femoral version [8].

Bone stock of the acetabulum is the first important issue for preoperative planning. If there is enough acetabular bone stock for implantation of the acetabular cup, it will facilitate the surgical process. But if there is not enough bone stock, then bone grafting and reconstruction systems for hip arthroplasty must be considered.

Anteversion of the femoral neck, femoral stenosis, and limb shortening are the main problems that can be faced. If the rotation of the affected extremity is advanced, corrective osteotomy can be planned [9, 10]. Femoral bowing is another difficulty in adaptation of the femoral component. Templating helps to select the ideal femoral component size.

5. Surgical approaches

Hip arthroplasty can be performed through anterolateral, anterior, and posterolateral approach. But extensile exposures are needed when there is difficulty in reaching the bone structures. Transtrochanteric approach is the one that can be used for this condition but nonunion is the most important complication. When femoral shortening is needed, a transfemoral approach and subtrochanteric osteotomy can be considered. There is an increased risk of sciatic nerve injury if leg lengthening is over 3–4 cm [11]. Femoral shortening osteotomy can be performed to avoid sciatic nerve injury [9].

6. Acetabular reconstruction

The aim of the acetabular reconstruction is to place the acetabular component to true acetabulum and to provide the normal biomechanical properties of the hip with normal hip center of rotation. Another important issue is the coverage of the acetabular cup with the acetabular bone. If there is not enough support with the bone, there can be increased stresses at the bone-implant (or bone-cement) interface, and mechanical failure can occur in the early period. For this reason, acetabular cup coverage by the natural bone must be done as much as possible. If acetabular cup coverage is not provided, alternative reconstructive techniques should be performed. The methods of reconstruction are discussed according to Crowe classification.

6.1. Crowe I hips (dysplasia)

These types of dysplastic hips have a minimal acetabular bony deformity. Reconstruction of the acetabulum can be done with the standard acetabular component. The component can be medialized to increase coverage of the implant by the natural bone. Good clinical results may be achieved using standard prosthesis stem sizes and press-fit acetabular component [12]. But small diameter femoral heads can be used for this reason that kinds of small implants must be ready to use in the operating room. Large femoral heads can be used when stability of acetabular component is achieved. Short-term results of large head metal-on-metal total hip arthroplasty in young and active patients with developmental dysplasia of the hip are similar to conventional THA [13]. Resurfacing hip arthroplasty is an option for the surgical treatment. There are several complications that can be seen like femoral neck fractures. But fixation of the acetabular component without adjuvant fixation can be achieved without complete acetabular coverage of the acetabular component [14].

6.2. Crowe II and III hips (low dislocation)

There is bone deficiency in the lateral part of the acetabulum. There is less bone support for the acetabular component. There are several surgical techniques to increase the coverage of the acetabular component. The medial wall of the acetabulum can be reamed deeper, so coverage of the acetabular component can be increased. But if the coverage of the cup is not suffi-

http://dx.doi.org/10.5772/67479

cient by this method, acetabular augmentation, reconstruction of the acetabulum in a superior location, or acetabular reinforcement rings are the other alternatives to provide coverage [15].

Bone grafts and cement are used for acetabular augmentation in the presence of superolateral acetabular defect. Allografts can be used, but patient's original femoral head is generally a good option. With this technique, normal hip center of rotation can be achieved with strong superolateral acetabular bone stock. A total of 60–70% coverage of the cementless acetabular cups can be acceptable [16, 17]. Long-term results of the bone stock of the acetabulum that was reconstructed using femoral head as autograft are favorable [18]. But if the amount of the acetabular component that is covered by graft is not large, there is a risk of graft resorption and collapse [19].

The other alternative technique is reconstruction of the acetabulum in a superior location which is called high hip center. The acetabular component is covered more with bone, and this technique facilitates biological fixation, and generally, there is no need for bone grafts. Main disadvantage of this technique is the need for small acetabular component with small femoral head which restricts range of motion of hip with abnormal hip biomechanics [20]. Midterm results of cementless acetabular component hip arthroplasty with high hip center are satisfactory with low rates of revision surgery [21].

Another technique is medialization of the acetabular component by over reaming the medial wall of the acetabulum. This technique was described first by Dunn and Hess [9]. It is also called acetabuloplasty. Medialization of the hip center of rotation increases coverage of the acetabular component and decreases joint reactive forces. Cup medialization has a compensatory effect on the femoral offset of the hip with less femoral antetorsion [22]. The only disadvantage of this method is the loss of bone stock of the medial acetabulum. The rate of medial protrusion of <60% is recommended for acceptable clinical and radiographic results [23].

The last technique is to use acetabular reinforcement rings for deficient acetabular bone. Ring is implanted to maximize host bone contact. Then, polyethylene cup is cemented in appropriate position for hip biomechanics. Reinforcement rings provide predictable good long-term results [24, 25].

6.3. Crowe IV hips (high dislocation)

In Crowe IV hips, the acetabulum is hypoplastic, but the superior rim of the acetabulum is less eroded than Crowe II and III hips, and bone stock is more than the Crowe II and III hips. Acetabular component can be placed to the anatomic hip center. But small-sized acetabular components can be used because of the hypoplastic acetabulum [26].

7. Femoral reconstruction

There are several deformities that can be seen in the femoral part of hip joint. There is an increased anteversion and valgus deformity. The medullar canal is generally narrower than normal medullar canal. Anterior-posterior diameter of the canal is more extensive than the medial-lateral diameter. The great trochanter can be placed posteriorly than normal hip.

7.1. Crowe I and II hips

In Crowe type I and type II dysplasias, femoral length is not a problem for reconstruction. Generally, there is no need for femoral osteotomy. Small diameter cemented or cementless stems can be used because of the narrower femoral medullar canal. Proximally coated femoral components are good options for the femoral reconstruction without osteotomy. Hip center of rotation can be changed in the reconstruction of acetabular part. For this reason, anteversion of the femoral component is an important issue for the hip stability. Placement of the femoral component is recommended in neutral or slight anteversion. Anteversion of the femoral neck can be significant in some hips, so femoral component anteversion must be aligned to the axis of the knee joint.

7.2. Crowe III and IV hips

After the center of hip rotation is configured in the true acetabulum, reduction of the hip joint in Crowe type III and IV hips is difficult because of the femoral length. Isolated soft tissue release is not enough for the reduction. For this reason, femoral osteotomies should be done. If the reduction of the hip joint is maintained after the soft tissue release, resulting in leg lengthening of more than 4 cm, then sciatic nerve injury may occur [27, 28].

There are two kinds of femoral osteotomies that can be performed in total hip arthroplasty for Crowe Types III and IV hips. First one is trochanteric osteotomy with proximal femoral shortening. Trochanteric osteotomy provides visualization of femur and acetabulum and preserves abductor mechanism with low risk of dislocation [29]. But risk of nonunion of great trochan-

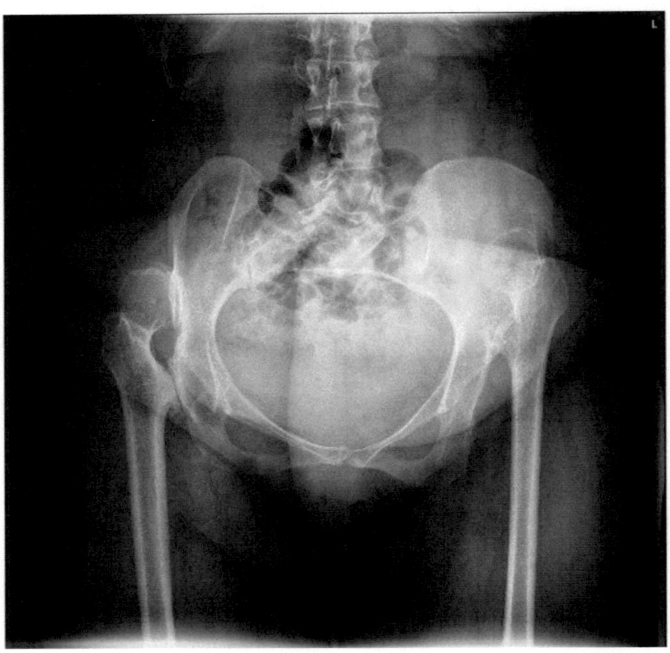

Figure 2. Bilateral Crowe IV developmental dysplasia of the hip. Both acetabula have bone deficiency with narrow femoral canal.

http://dx.doi.org/10.5772/67479

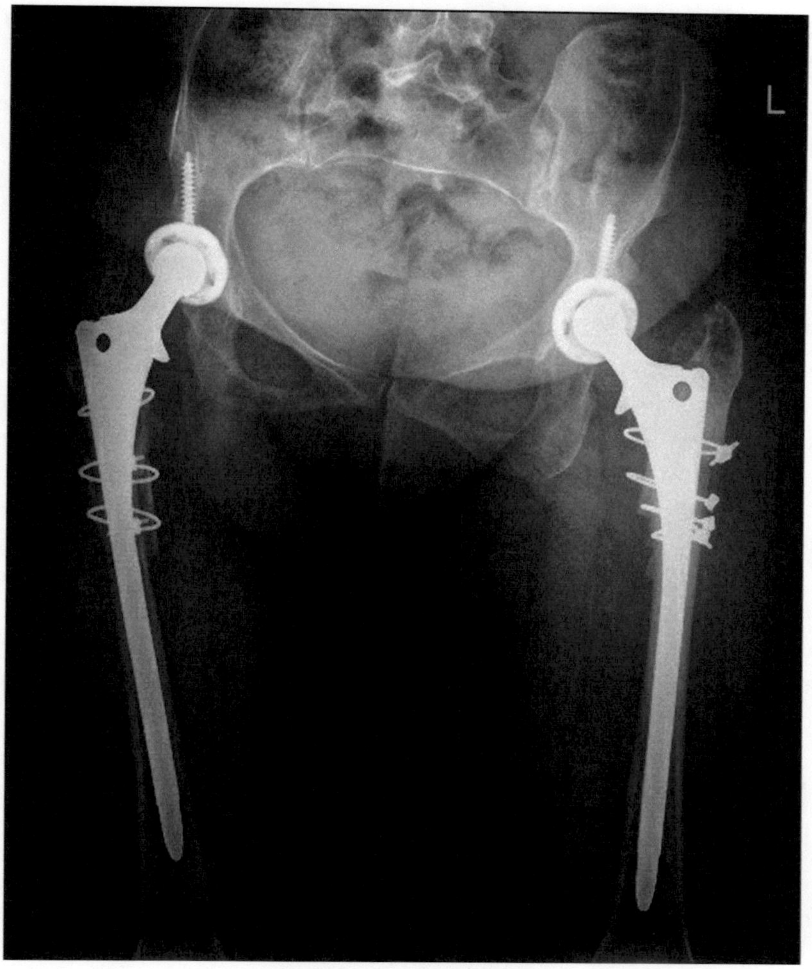

Figure 3. Postoperative radiograph of the pelvis showing bilateral reconstruction. Both acetabular reconstructions are done in a higher position than the true acetabulum because of the acetabular bone deficiency. Bilateral femoral shortening has been performed with usage of resected bone as auto graft.

ter is much with this technique [30, 31]. Subtrochanteric osteotomy preserves the metaphyseal region and has an advantage of correcting the rotational abnormalities with femoral shortening [32, 33]. After subtrochanteric femoral shortening, osteotomy noncemented femoral component can be used but a cemented DDH specific stem is preferable.

Subtrochanteric osteotomy is performed through a lateral approach than a transverse osteotomy is created in the subtrochanteric region. A femoral component is inserted to the proximal part of the osteotomy; then, hip is reduced. At this time, the amount of the femoral shortening can be calculated, and second cut is performed on distal part. Then, distal part of the femoral component is inserted to the distal fragment with adjusting anteversion. Prophylactic cerclage wiring of the fragments can prevent fractures. The resected portion of femur can be used as auto graft over the osteotomy line (**Figures 2** and **3**). Instead of a transverse osteotomy, a chevron-shaped osteotomy which was defined by Becker and Gustillo can be performed for more rotational stability [34].

In some cases, there can be an impingement of the trochanter on the pelvis in abduction or on the posterior acetabulum in external rotation. To solve impingement in abduction, trochanter is osteotomized and reattached distally. Trochanter is osteotomized and reattached laterally for the impingement in external rotation.

8. Bearing surfaces

Generally, there are three types of bearing surface alternatives for hip arthroplasty. Metal on polyethylene is the one that is used mostly. Polyethylene wear is the important issue for osteolysis and revision surgery. Most of the patients with DDH have to be performed hip arthroplasty in younger ages than the primary osteoarthritis. For this reason, other bearing surface alternatives must be chosen for the younger patients. Metal on metal bearing surface has an advantage of larger head sizes with small acetabular components. Larger head sizes provide more range of motion [35, 36]. Adverse allergic reactions and increased ion concentrations in the blood are the main unknown circumstances [37]. Ceramic on ceramic bearing surfaces has low friction but component fracture, development of noise, and less implant size options are the restrictive situations.

9. Total hip replacement in developmental dysplasia of the hip—pitfalls and challenges

9.1. Acetabular part

Cemented acetabular components can be used for the reconstruction of the acetabulum with the acetabular wall defects. Providing appropriate position of the component can be difficult because of the acetabular bone defects. Inappropriate placement of the acetabular cup causes decreased range of motion, less stability, and hip dislocation. Aseptic loosening is the main problem as a result of inappropriate placement of the acetabular cup in the long-term follow-up period. Cemented acetabular components have variable results in the literature. Survival ratio of the acetabular component was found 96% and 91% at 15 years with excellent long-term clinical and radiographic survivorship for acetabular dysplasia [38]. In another study with mean follow-up period of 15.7 year, the survival of the cemented acetabular component was 78%. The main reason of revision surgery was aseptic loosening with ratio of 88.3%. Higher rate of failure of the acetabular component was determined with increasing severity of hip dysplasia according to Crowe and Hartofilakidis classification [39]. Proximal migration of the hip center of rotation and nonanatomic placement of the acetabular component are the main reasons for aseptic loosening of the cemented acetabular component [40]. Nowadays, cemented acetabular reconstruction is not the first line treatment modality because of high revision rates [41, 42].

Coverage ratio of noncemented cups is the main important issue for the survival of the implant. For this reason, we must provide as much as possible surface coverage of the acetabular cup by acetabulum. But acetabular wall fracture can occur while reaming of the acetabulum. Reconstruction plates must be ready in the operating room. Noncemented acetabular components with grafts have same survival rates like the cemented acetabular components, with revision rates of 0–5% [43, 44]. The 20-year survivorship free from acetabular revision was 66% for noncemented acetabular components with femoral head as autograft [45]. In another study, 57% of the acetabular components underwent revision at a mean of 14.6 years because of osteolysis [46]. Twenty percent of the superolateral aspect of the acetabular cup could be left uncovered to prevent the failure risk [47] but there is no exact data about the amount of adequate acetabular cup coverage. Li et al reported results of the hip arthroplasty with more than 30% lateral uncoverage of noncemented acetabular components. There were no prosthesis revision and loosening during the mean 4.8 years follow-up [48]. Tikhilov et al. recommend acetabular component fixation without screws with moderate uncoverage within 25% but they offer two-screw fixation with significant uncoverage to 35% [49].

High hip center is another reconstruction option. The new acetabulum in the high hip center does not have strong osseous structures like true acetabulum. Reaming of the new acetabulum for the acetabular component can be resulted as a perforation of the bone. Superior wall of the acetabulum is not so strong, and acetabular cup stabilization cannot be sufficient. Acetabular cup stabilization can be provided with extra screws. These extra screws can cause neurovascular injury. In some cases, the new acetabulum can be formed in a higher position than the true acetabulum because of the acetabular bone deficiency (**Figure 2**). There are several studies that showed good results with cemented and noncemented acetabular components [21, 50, 51]. Results of a study that was compared the survivorship of the components for anatomical or high-cup placement; 100% in the anatomical placement and 97% for high hip center group [52]. Higher loosening and revision rates for both femoral and acetabular components have been reported with cemented acetabular cups for high hip center [40, 53]. There is a correlation between lateral displacement of the hip center and higher rates of component loosening [40].

Medialization of the acetabular cup can provide more surface coverage of the acetabular component by acetabular bone. To achieve a good stabilization, acetabular component can be 1 size larger than the acetabular reamer size. While impacting the acetabular component, there is a risk for acetabular fracture. If a fracture occurs, we must check the stability of the acetabular component. If the stability of the acetabular component is insufficient, stabilization must be maintained with extra acetabular cup screws. Medialization of the acetabular component by medial wall reaming has been reported low revision rates with both cemented and noncemented components [7, 54]. Medial wall defect of 25% of the acetabular area is recommended [54]. But in another study, higher loosening rates of the cemented components have been determined [55].

9.2. Femoral part

Narrower femoral canal in DDH is the main problem for femoral component. Cemented femoral components have an advantage of low fracture risk during the fixation. Cement mantle must cover one third of the cross-sectional area of the femoral canal. Distal centralizer must be used for the correct placement of the femoral component. Appropriate anteversion, valgus, and varus position of the femoral component must be provided in the period of cement polymerization. Modular or cemented stem should be used for extreme anteversion. Cemented femoral components have good long-term follow-up. Femoral component revision rates are 3–10% according to the literature [42, 56]. Cemented femoral component revision rates are lower than the cemented acetabular component. A total of 28 patients (35 hips) who underwent a cemented THA for DDH had been reviewed retrospectively. The overall revision rate was found 20%, and femoral revision rate was found 9% [57].

Noncemented femoral components are more popular nowadays. There is a risk of femur fracture while rasping the femoral canal and implantation of the noncemented femoral components. If a fracture occurs in that period, fixation must be achieved with cerclage wires or with a long femoral stem. Noncemented femoral component survival seems good. In a study of 15 patients with 17 hips, 57% underwent revision of the acetabular component at a mean of 14.6 years because of osteolysis. But no patient underwent revision because of femoral component loosening [46]. In another study with 106 patients with DDH, 18 acetabular revisions had been performed but there was no femoral component revision for any reason with mean follow-up period of 13.5 years [58]. Short-stem implants can be used for the reconstruction of the hip. Results of the hip arthroplasty with the short-stem implants in patients with DDH have good clinical outcome like primary osteoarthritis [59]. This type of implants can be used for lower grades of DDH.

Fixation of the subtrochanteric osteotomy with noncemented femoral components has favorable results. After the osteotomy and resection of the femoral segment, there can be inequality between proximal part cross-sectional area of the femoral canal and distal part cross-sectional area of the femoral canal. Long femoral stems improve stability. In some cases, modular femoral stems can be useful. Resected portion of femur can be used as auto graft over the osteotomy line. Also, this auto graft with cerclage wires has an additional support for stability (**Figure 3**). Crowe IV hips treated with subtrochanteric osteotomy using noncemented components show excellent healing rates [11, 60, 61]. But Park et al. reported three femoral nonunions on 24 hip arthroplasties with subtrochanteric shortening osteotomy [62].

There are several studies that compare THA outcomes in dysplastic and nondysplastic patients. As a result of a study which compares the dysplastic and nondysplastic hips, no significant difference was detected in Oxford Hip Score and revision rates between the two groups [63]. However, revision rates are more in dysplastic hips than in non-dysplastic hips in long-term follow-up [64]. Hip arthroplasty for DDH is complex surgery, and the cost of this procedure is more than a hip arthroplasty for primary osteoarthritis. Increased degree of dysplasia according to Crowe classification has been associated with higher costs [65].

10. Complications

Infection is an important complication that can occur after hip arthroplasty. The possibility of infection is increased in DDH. Surgical procedure time, exposure length, and use of more implants can be among the reasons. Nerve palsy, dislocation, and mechanical failure can be seen as a result of improper surgical technique and implant selection. Early loosening of the acetabular component, limping, and limb-length discrepancy can be seen in the high hip center type of reconstruction. Fracture and dislocation of the cup inside the pelvis are the most important complications for medialization technique. Nonunion of greater trochanter is an important complication after trochanteric osteotomy. Nonunion of the osteotomy site after femoral shortening procedures can be seen.

Author details

Özgür Korkmaz* and Melih Malkoç

*Address all correspondence to: ozkorkmaz00@yahoo.com

Department of Orthopedic and Traumatology, School of Medicine, Istanbul Medipol University, Turkey

References

[1] Argenson JN, Flecher X, Parratte S, Aubaniac JM: Anatomy of the dysplastic hip and consequences for total hip arthroplasty. Clin Orthop Relat Res. 2007;465:40–45. DOI: 10.1097/BLO.0b013e3181576052.

[2] Ito H, Matsuno T, Hirayama T, Tanino H, Yamanaka Y, Minami A: Three-dimensional computed tomography analysis of non-osteoarthritic adult acetabular dysplasia. Skeletal Radiol. 2009;38:131–139. DOI: 10.1007/s00256-008-0601-x.

[3] Sanchez-Sotelo J, Trousdale RT, Berry DJ, Cabanela ME: Surgical treatment of developmental dysplasia of the hip in adults: I. Nonarthroplasty options. J Am Acad Orthop Surg. 2002;10(5):321–333.

[4] Liu S, Zuo J, Li Z, Yang Y, Liu T, Xiao J, Gao Z: Study of three-dimensional morphology of the proximal femur in developmental adult dysplasia of the hip suggests that the on-shelf modular prosthesis may not be an ideal choice for patients with Crowe type IV hips. Int Orthop. 2016;14:1–7. DOI: 10.1007/s00264-016-3248-6.

[5] Liu R, Liang J, Wang K, Dang X, Bai C: Sciatic nerve course in adult patients with unilateral developmental dysplasia of the hip: implications for hip surgery. BMC Surg. 2015;31;15(1):1. DOI: 10.1186/1471-2482-15-14.

[6] Crowe JF, Mani VJ, Ranawat CS: Total hip replacement in congenital dislocation and dysplasia of the hip. J Bone Joint Surg Am. 1979;61(1):15–23.

[7] Hartofilakidis G, Stamos K, Karachalios T, Ioannidis TT, Zacharakis N: Congenital hip disease in adults. Classification of acetabular deficiencies and operative treatment with acetabuloplasty combined with total hip arthroplasty. J Bone Joint Surg Am. 1996;78(5):683–692.

[8] Kim JS, Park TS, Park SB, Kim JS, Kim IY, Kim SI: Measurement of femoral neck anteversion in 3D. Part 1: 3D imaging method. Med Biol Eng Comput. 2000;38:603–609.

[9] Dunn HK, Hess WE: Total hip reconstruction in chronically dislocated hips. J Bone Joint Surg Am. 1976;58:838–845.

[10] Kilicoglu OI, Turker M, Akgul T, Yazicioglu O: Cementless total hip arthroplasty with modified oblique femoral shortening osteotomy in Crowe type IV congenital hip dislocation. J Arthroplasty. 2013;28:117–125 DOI: 10.1016/j.arth.2012.06.014.

[11] Krych AJ, Howard JL, Trousdale RT, Cabanela ME, Berry DJ: Total hip arthroplasty with shortening subtrochanteric osteotomy in Crowe type-IV developmental dysplasia. J Bone Joint Surg Am. 2009;91:2213–2221. DOI: 10.2106/JBJS. H.01024.

[12] Bożek M, Bielecki T, Nowak R, Żelawski M: Arthroplasty in patients with congenital hip dysplasia—early evaluation of a treatment method. Ortop Traumatol Rehabil. 2013;15(1):49–59. DOI: 10.5604/15093492.1032794.

[13] Yalcin N, Kilicarslan K, Cicek H, Kayaalp C, Yildirim H: Crowe type I and II DDH managed by large diameter metal-on-metal total hip arthroplasty. Hip Int. 2011;21(2):168–175. DOI: 10.5301/HIP.2011.7418.

[14] Amstutz HC, Antoniades JT, Le Duff MJ: Results of metal-on-metal hybrid hip resurfacing for Crowe type-I and II developmental dysplasia. J Bone Joint Surg Am. 2007;89(2):339–346. DOI: 10.2106/JBJS.F.00576.

[15] Dapuzzo MR, Sierra RJ: Acetabular considerations during total hip arthroplasty for hip dysplasia. Orthop Clin North Am. 2012;43(3):369–375. DOI: 10.1016/j.ocl.2012.05.012.

[16] Paavilainen T, Hoikka V, Solonen KA: Cementless total replacement for severely dysplastic or dislocated hips. J Bone Joint Surg Br. 1990;72:205–211.

[17] Shen B, Yang J, Wang L, Zhou ZK, Kang PD, Pei FX: Midterm results of hybrid total hip arthroplasty for treatment of osteoarthritis secondary to developmental dysplasia of the hip-Chinese experience. J Arthroplasty. 2009;24:1157–1163. DOI: 10.1016/j.arth.2009.07.002.

[18] Farrell CM, Berry DJ, Cabanela ME: Autogenous femoral head bone grafts for acetabular deficiency in total-hip arthroplasty for developmental dysplasia of the hip: long-term effect on pelvic bone stock. J Arthroplasty. 2005;20(6):698–702. DOI: 10.1016/j.arth.2004.11.004.

[19] Mulroy RD, Harris WH: Failure of acetabular autogenous grafts in total hip arthroplasty. Increasing incidence: a follow-up note. J Bone Joint Surg Am. 1990;72(10):1536–1540.

[20] Komiyama K, Nakashima Y, Hirata M, Hara D, Kohno Y, Iwamoto Y: Does high hip center decrease range of motion in total hip arthroplasty? A computer simulation study. J Arthroplasty. 2016;15. DOI: 10.1016/j.arth.2016.03.014.

[21] Chen M, Luo ZL, Wu KR, Zhang XQ, Ling XD, Shang XF: Cementless total hip arthroplasty with a high hip center for hartofilakidis type B developmental dysplasia of the hip: results of midterm follow-up. J Arthroplasty. 2016;31(5):1027–1034. DOI: 10.1016/j.arth.2015.11.009.

[22] Terrier A, Levrero Florencio F, Rüdiger HA: Benefit of cup medialization in total hip arthroplasty is associated with femoral anatomy. Clin Orthop Relat Res. 2014;472(10):3159–3165. DOI: 10.1007/s11999-014-3787-3.

[23] Zha GC, Sun JY, Guo KJ, Zhao FC, Pang Y, Zheng X: Medial protrusio technique in cementless total hip arthroplasty for developmental dysplasia of the hip: a prospective 6- to 9-year follow-up of 43 consecutive patients. J Arthroplasty. 2016;31. DOI: 10.1016/j.arth.2016.01.052.

[24] Ewers A, Spross C, Ebneter L, Külling F, Giesinger K, Zdravkovic V, Erhardt J: 10-year survival of acetabular reinforcement rings/cages for complex hip arthroplasty. Open Orthop J. 2015;159:163–167. DOI: 10.2174/1874325001509010163.

[25] Sadri H, Pfander G, Siebenrock KA, Tannast M, Koch P, Fujita H, Ballmer P, Ganz R: Acetabular reinforcement ring in primary total hip arthroplasty: a minimum 10-year follow-up. Arch Orthop Trauma Surg. 2008;128(8):869–877. DOI: 10.1007/s00402-008-0612-z.

[26] Li W, Zhang W, Bai G, Huang Z, Shen R: Total hip arthroplasty for treatment of Crowe type IV congenital dysplasia of hip with dislocation in adults. Zhongguo Xiu Fu Chong Jian Wai Ke Za Zhi. 2013;27(10):1153–1156.

[27] Farrell CM, Springer BD, Haidukewych GJ, Morrey BF: Motor nerve palsy following primary total hip arthroplasty. J Bone Joint Surg Am. 2005;87:2619–2625. DOI: 10.2106/JBJS.C.01564.

[28] Eggli S, Hankemayer S, Müller ME: Nerve palsy after leg lengthening in total replacement arthroplasty for developmental dysplasia of the hip. J Bone Joint Surg Br. 1999;81:843–845.

[29] Kerboull L, Hamadouche M, Kerboull M: Transtrochanteric approach to the hip. Interact Surg. 2007;2:149–154.

[30] Menon PC, Griffiths WE, Hook WE, Higgins B: Trochanteric osteotomy in total hip arthroplasty: comparison of 2 techniques. J Arthroplasty. 1998;13:92–96.

[31] Kerboull M, Hamadouche M, Kerboull L: Total hip arthroplasty for Crowe type IV developmental hip dysplasia: a long-term follow-up study. J Arthroplasty. 2001;16:170–176.

[32] Chareancholvanich K, Becker DA, Gustilo RB: Treatment of congenital dislocated hip by arthroplasty with femoral shortening. Clin Orthop Relat Res. 1999;360:127–135.

[33] Yasgur DJ, Stuchin SA, Adler EM, DiCesare PE: Subtrochanteric femoral shortening osteotomy in total hip arthroplasty for high-riding developmental dislocation of the hip. J Arthroplasty. 1997;12(8):880–888.

[34] Becker DA, Gustilo RB: Double-chevron subtrochanteric shortening derotational femoral osteotomy combined with total hip arthroplasty for the treatment of complete congenital dislocation of the hip in the adult. Preliminary report and description of a new surgical technique. J Arthroplasty. 1995;10(3):313–318.

[35] Schmalzried TP, Peters PC, Maurer BT, Bragdon CR, Harris WH: Long duration metal-on-metal total hip arthroplasties with low wear of the articulating surfaces. J Arthroplasty. 1996;11:322.

[36] Sieber HP, Rieker CB, Kottig P. Analysis of 118 second-generation metal-on-metal retrieved hip implants: J Bone Joint Surg Br. 1999;81(1):46–50.

[37] Willert HG, Buchhorn GH, Fayyazi A, Flury R, Windler M, Köster G, Lohmann CH: Metal-on-metal bearings and hypersensitivity in patients with artificial hip joints. A clinical and histomorphological study. J Bone Joint Surg Am. 2005;87:280. DOI: 10.2106/JBJS.A.02039pp.

[38] Akiyama H, Kawanabe K, Iida H, Haile P, Goto K, Nakamura T: Long-term results of cemented total hip arthroplasty in developmental dysplasia with acetabular bulk bone grafts after improving operative techniques. J Arthroplasty. 2010;25(5):716–720. DOI: 10.1016/j.arth.2009.05.017.

[39] Chougle A, Hemmady MV, Hodgkinson JP: Severity of hip dysplasia and loosening of the socket in cemented total hip replacement. A long-term follow-up. J Bone Joint Surg Br. 2005;87(1):16–20.

[40] Stans AA, Pagnano MW, Shaughnessy WJ, Hanssen AD: Results of total hip arthroplasty for Crowe type III developmental hip dysplasia. Clin Orthop Relat Res. 1998;348:149–157.

[41] MacKenzie JR, Kelley SS, Johnston RC: Total hip replacement for coxarthrosis secondary to congenital dysplasia and dislocation of the hip. Long-term results. J Bone Joint Surg Am. 1996;78:55–61.

[42] Numair J, Joshi AB, Murphy JC, Porter ML, Hardinge K: Total hip arthroplasty for congenital dysplasia or dislocation of the hip. survivorship analysis and long-term results. J Bone Joint Surg Am. 1997;79:1352–1360.

[43] Morsi E, Garbuz D, Gross AE: Total hip arthroplasty with shelf grafts using noncemented cups. A long-term follow-up. J Arthroplasty. 1996;11(1):81–85.

[44] Silber DA, Engh CA: Cementless total hip arthroplasty with femoral head bone grafting for hip dysplasia. J Arthroplasty. 1990;5:231–240.

[45] Abdel MP, Stryker LS, Trousdale RT, Berry DJ, Cabanela ME: Noncemented acetabular components with femoral head autograft for acetabular reconstruction in developmental dysplasia of the hip: a concise follow-up report at a mean of twenty years. J Bone Joint Surg Am. 2014;96(22):1878–1882. DOI: 10.2106/JBJS.N.00061.

[46] Imbuldeniya AM, Walter WL, Zicat BA, Walter WK: Cementless total hip replacement without femoral osteotomy in patients with severe developmental dysplasia of the hip: minimum 15-year clinical and radiological results. Bone Joint J. 2014;96–B(11):1449–1454. DOI: 10.1302/0301-620X.96B11.33698.

[47] Garvin KL, Bowen MK, Salvati EA, Ranawat CS: Long-term results of total hip arthroplasty in congenital dislocation and dysplasia of the hip. A follow-up note. J Bone Joint Surg Am. 1991;73:1348–1354.

[48] Li H, Mao Y, Oni JK, Dai K, Zhu Z: Total hip replacement for developmental dysplasia of the hip with more than 30% lateral uncoverage of noncemented acetabular components. Bone Joint J. 2013;95–B(9):1178–1183. DOI: 10.1302/0301-620X.95B9.31398.

[49] Tikhilov R, Shubnyakov I, Burns S, Shabrov N, Kuzin A, Mazurenko A, Denisov A: Experimental study of the installation acetabular component with uncoverage in arthroplasty patients with severe developmental hip dysplasia. Int Orthop. 2015;40:1–5. DOI: 10.1007/s00264-015-2951-z.

[50] Russotti GM, Harris WH: Proximal placement of the acetabular component in total hip arthroplasty. A long-term follow-up study. J Bone Joint Surg Am. 1991;73(4):587–592.

[51] Schutzer SF, Harris WH: High placement of porous-coated acetabular components in complex total hip arthroplasty. J Arthroplasty. 1994;9(4):359–367.

[52] Murayama T, Ohnishi H, Okabe S, Tsurukami H, Mori T, Nakura N, Uchida S, Sakai A, Nakamura T: 15-year comparison of cementless total hip arthroplasty with anatomical or high cup placement for Crowe I to III hip dysplasia. Orthopedics. 2012;35(3):e313–e318. DOI: 10.3928/01477447-20120222-28.

[53] Pagnano W, Hanssen AD, Lewallen DG, Shaughnessy WJ: The effect of superior placement of the acetabular component on the rate of loosening after total hip arthroplasty. J Bone Joint Surg Am. 1996;78(7):1004–1014.

[54] Dorr LD, Tawakkol S, Moorthy M, Long W, Wan Z: Medial protrusio technique for placement of a porous-coated, hemispherical acetabular component withoutcement in a total hip arthroplasty in patients who have acetabular dysplasia. J Bone Joint Surg Am. 1999;81(1):83–92.

[55] Hartofilakidis G, Georgiades G, Babis GC, Yiannakopoulos CK: Evaluation of two surgical techniques for acetabular reconstruction in total hip replacement for congenital hip disease: results after a minimum 10-year follow-up. J Bone Joint Surg Br. 2008;90(6):724–730. DOI: 10.1302/0301-620X.90B6.20490.

[56] Sochart DH, Porter ML: The long-term results of Charnley low-friction arthroplasty in young patients who have congenital dislocation, degenerative osteoarthrosis, or rheumatoid arthritis. J Bone Joint Surg Am. 1997;79(11):1599–1617.

[57] Howie CR, Ohly NE, Miller B: Cemented total hip arthroplasty with subtrochanteric osteotomy in dysplastic hips. Clin Orthop Relat Res. 2010;468(12):3240–3247. DOI: 10.1007/s11999-010-1367-8.

[58] Kaneuji A, Sugimori T, Ichiseki T, Fukui K, Takahashi E, Matsumoto T: Cementless anatomic total hip femoral component with circumferential porous coating for hips with developmental dysplasia: a minimum 10-year follow-up period. J Arthroplasty. 2013;28(10):1746–1750. DOI: 10.1016/j.arth.2013.06.030.

[59] Budde S, Floerkemeier T, Thorey F, Ezechieli M, Claassen L, Ettinger M, Bredow J, Windhagen H, Lewinski GV: A short-stem hip implant with metaphyseal anchorage in patients with developmental dysplasia of the hip. Technol Health Care. 2016;59: 559–569. DOI: 10.3233/THC-161151.

[60] Bernasek TL, Haidukewych GJ, Gustke KA, Hill O, Levering M: Total hip arthroplasty requiring subtrochanteric osteotomy for developmental hip dysplasia: 5- to 14-year results. J Arthroplasty. 2007;22:145–150. DOI: 10.1016/j.arth.2007.05.014.

[61] Ollivier M, Abdel MP, Krych AJ, Trousdale RT, Berry DJ: Long-term results of total hip arthroplasty with shortening subtrochanteric osteotomy in Crowe IV developmental dysplasia. J Arthroplasty. 31. DOI: 10.1016/j.arth.2016.01.049.

[62] Park MS, Kim KH, Jeong WC: Transverse subtrochanteric shortening osteotomy in primary total hip arthroplasty for patients with severe hip developmental dysplasia. J Arthroplasty. 2007;22(7):1031–1036. DOI: 10.1016/j.arth.2007.05.011.

[63] Boyle MJ, Frampton CM, Crawford HA: Early results of total hip arthroplasty in patients with developmental dysplasia of the hip compared with patients with osteoarthritis. J Arthroplasty. 2012;27(3):386–390. DOI: 10.1016/j.arth.2011.06.024.

[64] Engesaeter LB, Furnes O, Havelin LI: Developmental dysplasia of the hip—good results of later total hip arthroplasty: 7135 primary total hip arthroplasties after developmental dysplasia of the hip compared with 59774 total hip arthroplasties in idiopathic coxarthrosis followed for 0 to 15 years in the Norwegian Arthroplasty Register. J Arthroplasty. 2008;23(2):235–240. DOI: 10.1016/j.arth.2007.03.023.

[65] Ashraf A, Larson AN, Maradit-Kremers H, Kremers WK, Lewallen DG: Hospital costs of total hip arthroplasty for developmental dysplasia of the hip. Clin Orthop Relat Res. 2014;472(7):2237–2244. DOI: 10.1007/s11999-014-3587-9.